GRANGER WESTBERG, AUTHOR OF *GOOD GRIEF*

*'Both informative and practical...
to be commended for her sensitivity
and thoroughness.'*

JOSEPH CARDINAL BERNARDIN, ARCHBISHOP
OF CHICAGO, CARER TO HIS MOTHER

*'An honest and loving book written by
a person who is very familiar... with
the dilemmas and challenges facing
sufferers, carers and their families.'*

DR PENNY STANWAY, DOCTOR, JOURNALIST
AND AUTHOR OF *THE NATURAL GUIDE TO
WOMEN'S HEALTH*

SHARON FISH MOONEY teaches nursing research and gerontology on-line at Indiana Wesleyan University and Regis University, Denver, Colorado, USA. She has a PhD from the University of Rochester in New York and has taught courses on Parish Nursing at McMaster Divinity College, Canada. Sharon co-authored a classic nursing textbook on spiritual care and is a freelance writer and conference speaker. The experiences of caring for her own mother through Alzheimer's and her nursing experience on special care units for older people with dementia have greatly informed this book.

*To LaVonne Neff and Morag Reeve,
who helped birth this book in the US
and the UK, and to all those who cared
and shared their lives with me.*

ALZHEIMER'S

CARING FOR YOUR LOVED ONE, CARING FOR YOURSELF

Sharon Fish Mooney

LION

A Lion Book
an imprint of
Lion Hudson plc
Wilkinson House, Jordan Hill Road,
Oxford OX2 8DR, England
www.lionhudson.com
ISBN 978 0 7459 5289 5

First (US) edition 1990
First (UK) edition 1991
This edition 2008
10 9 8 7 6 5 4 3 2 1 0

Acknowledgements
pp. 9, 17, 212 Scripture quotations taken from the Revised Standard
Version of the Bible, © 1946, 1952, 1971 by the Division of Christian
Education of the National Council of Churches of Christ in the USA,
and used by permission.

pp. 82, 162 Scripture quotations taken from Today's English Version
(The Good News Bible), © 1966, 1971, 1976, 1992 by the American
Bible Society. Used by permission.

pp. 128, 184 Scripture quotations taken from the *Holy Bible,
New International Version*, copyright © 1973, 1978, 1984
International Bible Society. Used by permission of Zondervan
and Hodder & Stoughton Limited. All rights reserved. The 'NIV'
and 'New International Version' trademarks are registered in the
United States Patent and Trademark Office by International Bible
Society. Use of either trademark requires the permission of
International Bible Society. UK trademark number 1448790.

This book has been printed on paper and board independently
certified as having been produced from sustainable forests.

A catalogue record for this book is available
from the British Library

Typeset in 9/12pt ITC Century BT
Printed and bound in Wales
by Creative Print and Design

Acknowledgements

My hope for all who read this book is that you will be encouraged. You are not alone as you reach out to care for your loved ones.

I am deeply grateful to Jack Fisher, Kathleen Fisher Poling, Marian Gierasch and Mary Butts, four carers who formed the original Alzheimer's support group in Oneonta, New York, USA, and who faithfully kept the candle burning in monthly meetings for those who needed help and encouragement.

Special thanks to Mary Johnson, who read the original manuscript, and to the dozens of carers who were willing to share their experiences for others to learn from, including me. To protect carers' privacy, no names are included and, in some instances, certain identifying details have been changed at their request. Scenarios that introduce various chapters weave together all our stories, our fears, our hopes, our feelings. The people described could well be your mother or father, husband or wife, sister or brother, son or daughter.

I want to thank Dr Raymond Vickers, M.D., who was medical director of the New York State Veterans' Home, Oxford, New York; he read and edited the original manuscript with a physician's eye. Special thanks also to his wife, Barbara, who gave generously of her time and talents to encourage carers for many years in a variety of settings.

Thank you to the following people who lovingly cared for my mother in our home or theirs over the years: Sylvia Davisson, Pat Gifford, Janet Roseboom, Bunny Rodriquez, Kim Lund, Carol Rose, Katie Jenison and Debbie Derry. Thanks to the staff at Stamford Nursing Home in Stamford, New York, who cared for my mother as if she were *their* mother during the final days of her life. And thank you to the staff and friends of Inter County Home Care, who were always there when I needed them.

I would also like to acknowledge the special care unit at Kirkhaven, Rochester, New York, where I worked; the Rochester, New York, chapter of the Alzheimer's Association; and Dr Eric G. Tangalos, Mayo Clinic Alzheimer's Disease Center, Rochester, Minnesota, for their helpful assistance.

Special thanks to the following for a number of reasons: Dr Steven Szebenyi and Dr Donald Pollock from Bassett Hospital, Cooperstown, New York, who helped me over the years with medical management;

Emalene Shepherd of the Writer's Digest School, who watered a vision that began with a carers' column; and Morag Reeve and Kate Kirkpatrick, editors at Lion Hudson, who wanted to keep this book in print.

I especially want to acknowledge and thank Susan Cuthbert, my editor at Lion who originally anglicized this book, incorporating information about the British health-care system, and Jan Dewing from the UK Wandering Network for her valuable updated information for this current edition. My final thanks go to the many friends who prayed for and encouraged me and to my husband Scott and stepson Richard, who show constant care for me.

I am grateful.

SHARON FISH MOONEY

Acknowledgements from the UK editor

With grateful thanks to Clive Evers for the benefit of his special knowledge. Also to Mrs Joan King and the Oxfordshire Branch of the Alzheimer's Society, to my friends Janet Hathaway, Mari-an Watkins, Janet Baraclough, Sarah Moore, Bridget Banks and Dr Peter Garside, and to my mother-in-law Mrs Hazel Cuthbert, for their help with the finer details of the 'anglicization'. It has been much appreciated, though of course responsibility for any deficiencies rests firmly with me.

SUSAN CUTHBERT

Contents

Something Has Gone Wrong

A bruised reed he will not break,
and a dimly burning wick
he will not quench.

THE BOOK OF ISAIAH

Chapter One

Bruised Reeds and Dimly Burning Wicks

Muriel sat down at the kitchen table and slowly buttered her toast. Fifteen minutes of silence, twenty if she was lucky. Quiet time alone to enjoy the toast, a cup of coffee, and a quick read through the morning paper before the real work began: getting her mother up, washed, fed, toileted, walked and dressed for the day. And then, later in the morning, several loads of laundry including her mother's urine-stained sheets.

'Bye, Mum,' Susan shouted as she grabbed her books and headed out of the door to catch the school bus.

'Bye,' yelled Bruce, scooping up his rucksack and racing past his sister.

Muriel glanced out of the window and caught a glimpse of the bus as it rounded the curve and disappeared out of sight beyond the hedgerow.

The school term would be over in a few weeks. Unfortunately, Muriel knew the children weren't looking forward to being home all summer. When she'd asked them they said they didn't mind, but her neighbour had told her the truth. When the neighbour had asked Susan how she was going to spend her summer holiday, Susan had just shrugged her shoulders and looked unhappy. And Bruce said, 'We aren't going anywhere because of Grandma.'

'Mur. Mur.'

'Ten of my twenty minutes wasted thinking about something I can't do anything about,' Muriel thought.

'Mur. Mur.'

'In a minute, Mother,' Muriel called back, hastily swallowing the last of the coffee, running her plate under the tap and shoving it into the dishwasher.

Ruth. Muriel's mother. Ruth was the reason the children weren't looking forward to their summer holiday.

Muriel couldn't blame them. It wasn't easy being thirteen and seven and having a grandparent with Alzheimer's disease living with you twenty-four hours a day. A grandmother who didn't do the things grandmothers were supposed to do – like tell you what adorable grandchildren you were, listen to your stories and bake you biscuits. A grandmother who, instead, sometimes threatened you and didn't even know your name, babbled incoherently at times, and had almost burned your house down trying to boil an egg.

Muriel's father had died fifteen years earlier, and her mother never remarried. Ruth continued to live alone in the old family farmhouse, three miles from Muriel, Carl and the children. At age sixty-five, Ruth had begun to show signs of memory loss, but the signs were so subtle that Muriel had hardly noticed them.

Her mother was for ever losing things: her glasses, her cheque book, her keys. When Muriel would drop in unexpectedly she'd often find Ruth rummaging through drawers, muttering under her breath. But then, for as long as Muriel could remember, her mother had misplaced things.

Then her mother stopped remembering.

Birthdays were first. Muriel's. Carl's. Susan's. Bruce's. Her own. Very unlike the mother who had never failed to send a card, buy a present or bake a cake.

Appointments were next. The dentist, hairdresser, chiropodist – all were forgotten. Muriel had calls from all three of them one month asking where Ruth was.

Muriel's mother had notes posted all over the house. 'Memory joggers,' Ruth called them. But she still forgot.

And then there were names. Odd, Muriel had thought, that her mother couldn't seem to remember the names of the children one Sunday when she was over for dinner. Ruth kept calling them Sally and Ron, the names of her own sister and brother. The children thought it was a game Grandma was playing. Muriel wasn't so sure.

It was Muriel's husband, Carl, who first realized there was more wrong with Ruth than simple age-related memory loss.

Carl stopped by the farm one morning to get Ruth's grocery list and found his mother-in-law taking a nap in a smoke-filled house. She had put a fruit cake in the oven, turned the oven on high and gone to sleep. The smoke detector was working, but Ruth had removed her hearing aid and, as she told them later, had forgotten where she put it. A look in the kitchen cupboards revealed more black-bottomed cake tins and saucepans, ample evidence that cooking was one task Ruth could no longer accomplish safely.

The final straw came several weeks later when Muriel got a phone call. Ruth was at the post office in town, having walked for two miles in the rain. She insisted she was in the bank, wanted to see the balance on her account, and demanded her money. Could Muriel please come and get her mother, asked the postmistress.

Muriel did. She got Ruth, took her home to the farm and started packing.

Moving hadn't been easy. Ruth became even more confused and disoriented in the new environment. She accused Muriel and Carl of stealing her money and selling the family farm.

The children, then aged ten and four, were a mixed blessing as far as Ruth was concerned. Sometimes she showered them with affection, and they basked in the attention. At other times they were also part of the supposed conspiracy to confiscate her property.

Bruce seemed to go with the flow of Grandma's mood swings, but Susan, who had known the love of a more stable grandmother, had a difficult time accepting the bizarre behaviour patterns that emerged. When Ruth had one of her verbal outbursts, Susan would run to her own room and stay there until her mother or father assured her the coast was clear.

Now, three years later, Ruth's paranoia was gone, but Susan's habit of retreat remained. Muriel hoped Susan would outgrow it. And she wished she didn't feel so guilty about the children.

'Mur. Mur,' Ruth called from the bedroom, the room Susan had given up when her grandmother moved in.

'Coming, Mother,' Muriel called, as she dried her hands on the tea towel and turned to go upstairs.

Alzheimer's: A Family Affair

This book is certainly not the first word on Alzheimer's disease, nor will it be the last. Rather it is one voice in a chorus speaking out about a devastating illness affecting the daily lives of millions of people worldwide. People like Muriel and Ruth. People like my mother and your mother, our fathers, husbands, wives, children. The cared for and the carers. The loved ones and those who love.

I am a writer, a registered nurse and a teacher. I have also been a carer. Over thirty years of hospital, nursing home and home-nursing experience have brought me in contact with many other carers and their loved ones. But my own mother brought the reality of Alzheimer's home. In 1980 she was diagnosed with senile dementia of the Alzheimer's type, and I was able to experience caregiving firsthand for over ten years, from the time I first moved home to help my father cope until her death in a nursing home. In 1989 I decided it was time to write about the things my mother was teaching me and the things I was learning from other carers.

After my mother's death I both worked and volunteered in a number of special care dementia units in the United States and Canada. This book tells the story of Alzheimer's from the varying perspectives of my life and work.

The scenarios that introduce various chapters in this book are based on the lives of many carers including myself. In them I've tried to weave together experiences, reminiscences and feelings to paint a picture of what Alzheimer's is really like.

This book is primarily for carers like myself – those who live with loved ones, visit them in nursing homes and various types of sheltered and residential care facilities, or show care and concern from afar. I also hope it will be of value to professional and voluntary carers who recognize illness as a family affair. And, too, I wrote it for friends. Without them, caring would be a very lonely experience.

In addition to drawing from my own experience and current research and literature, I interviewed dozens of carers who gave me permission to quote them. This gave direction for chapter topics and helped me focus on some primary concerns. The inclusion of appendices was designed with the professional carer in mind and for family carers wanting additional sources of more detailed information about current research and medication.

Whenever people talk about Alzheimer's, certain questions come up:

• How can I tell if my loved one has Alzheimer's? What are the early signs and symptoms?

• What causes Alzheimer's disease? Is it hereditary?

• How can I be sure my friend or relative is getting an accurate diagnosis? What's involved in the diagnostic process?

• What are some of the bizarre and bewildering behaviours peculiar to Alzheimer's disease? How can I manage them?

• Is there any specific treatment or cure?

• What's the purpose of all this suffering?

• How can I meet my own needs as a wife, husband, daughter, son?

• Is it normal for me to feel angry, guilty, depressed or resentful? How can I deal with these emotions?

• How can I deal with my loved one's physical needs?

• What kinds of resources are available to help care for my loved one at home? How can I find and pay for this care?

• How can a person decide to place a loved one in a nursing home? Is there ever a right time?

• Are brain post-mortems important? How can I find out about them?

• What will death be like for my loved one? What will my loved one's death be like for me?

We will look at each of these questions in detail in later chapters. But first, what is Alzheimer's? Who gets it?

Some Facts About Alzheimer's

Alzheimer's disease is a chronic, progressive, irreversible brain disorder or dementia for which there is no one definable cause, no definitive treatment and, to date, no foreseeable cure. The basic definition has remained the same over the years, though medical and social science research continues to hold out hope for the future as well as for the present generation of sufferers and their carers concerning ways to improve quality of life. This includes a number of approved medications and also specific behavioural interventions, a number of which have been the subject of research.

Dementia, the broader diagnostic category of which Alzheimer's is the primary type, is a multifaceted decline of intellectual functions of sufficient severity to interfere with an individual's activities of daily living, career, social relationships and social activities. Dementia involves personality changes, loss of memory and judgement, and difficulty with abstract thinking and orientation.

The word *dementia* literally means 'mind away' or 'deprived of mind'. Dementing illnesses are the result of one or more disease processes that can drastically alter people's behaviour and gradually bankrupt their minds and the lives of entire families. Alzheimer's disease is thought to be the primary cause of incurable dementia for men and women over the age of sixty-five, compared with other types of dementia. It is more common in women than in men.

According to the document *Dementia UK*, a comprehensive report published by the Alzheimer's Society (2007) produced by King's College London and the London School of Economics, conservative estimates are that up to 700,000 people in the UK suffer from some form of dementia. This translates to one in every eighty-eight people in the entire population, one in every six people over the age of eighty and one in fourteen people over the age of sixty-five. The consensus figures for 2005 from Alzheimer's Disease International estimated that over 24 million people may suffer from dementia in the world at large; this estimate could exceed 80 million by 2040.

Although Alzheimer's usually occurs after a person reaches the mid-sixties, with a significant increase after the age of eighty,

Alzheimer's can also afflict people in their forties and fifties. Though early-onset Alzheimer's is much rarer, it's not just a disease of the old or very old.

It is estimated that by 2025 the number of people suffering from dementia in the UK could be over one million. The accompanying emotional and economic costs stagger the imagination. Current total costs for dementia care in the UK for people over the age of sixty-five are estimated at between £17 billion and £18 billion per annum according to the Alzheimer's Society; this includes the caring contributions made by family members and friends. While the majority of people with dementia continue to live in a home environment supported by friends, relatives and community services, dementia sufferers currently fill nearly 67 per cent of all nursing home beds and over 52 per cent of residential care beds. Sixty thousand deaths per year are directly attributable to dementia: approximately 10 per cent of deaths in males over the age of sixty-five and 15 per cent in women of a comparable age.[1]

A leading cause of death in people older than seventy-five, Alzheimer's was called 'the disease of the twentieth century', a phrase attributed to writer and scientist Dr Lewis Thomas. It may well be the disease of the twenty-first century as well, as the over eighty-five population doubles.

Alzheimer's disease has also been described in the literature by carers as 'a funeral that never ends', 'a nightmare from which you never wake up', 'another name for madness', 'the silent epidemic', 'the slow death of the mind'. One of the most popular and practical books ever written on the subject of Alzheimer's disease, titled *The 36-Hour Day*,[2] reflects the reality of life for most carers.

Caring for a loved one with a dementing illness *does* seem to require more than seven days a week, twenty-four hours a day, sixty minutes an hour; the difficulties inherent in caring for someone with Alzheimer's disease are all too real.

But the difficulties are not the whole picture. Caring can also be an opportunity for growth. It can make us more patient, more compassionate, and more courageous people.

A beautiful verse in the Bible reads, 'A bruised reed he will not break, and a dimly burning wick he will not quench' (Isaiah 42:3). There is hope for the carer who feels battered and bruised in the battle against Alzheimer's disease. We need not be broken.

There is also hope for our loved ones, no matter how bizarre or bewildering their behaviour may be. As carers, we have daily opportunities to fan the flames of their hearts and spirits as we care for them in love.

And, it is hoped, our own hearts and spirits will be lifted up and comforted in the very process of caring as we discover untapped, unrecognized strengths in ourselves and in the people around us.

Chapter Two

Searching for the Truth

'I think my mother has Alzheimer's,' a friend confided to me over the phone one night. 'She has all the symptoms your mother does. She's confused and forgetful. She can't even remember her own name or mine, and she's having a lot of personality changes.'

'How long has this been going on?' I asked, puzzled, because this was the first time my friend had mentioned her mother's changing behaviour.

'Just about a month,' she said.

I told my friend her mother's condition might *not* be the more gradually developing disease of Alzheimer's and encouraged her to take her mother to a doctor immediately.

My friend's mother was diagnosed a short time later. She didn't have Alzheimer's. She had a rapidly growing brain tumour.

In past decades, Alzheimer's was one of the most underdiagnosed diseases. Today it has burst out of obscurity to become one of the most overdiagnosed, particularly among friends and family members who have read a lot about it in the popular literature.

Even some health-care professionals are guilty of making the instant diagnosis. Unfortunately, it's still not uncommon to hear carers say, 'My husband's doctor took one look at him and said, "He has all the symptoms of Alzheimer's. It's not necessary to run any tests."'

Yet brain post-mortem reports have indicated that some people actually diagnosed with Alzheimer's did not in fact have Alzheimer's. They showed none of Alzheimer's characteristic physical changes in the brain, even though they had exhibited symptoms of brain dementia. (Characteristic physical changes include senile plaques and neurofibrillary tangles that form in the brain tissue of people with Alzheimer's.)[1]

Alzheimer's is not the *only* disease process that causes dementia. There are also dozens of disorders whose symptoms can mimic those of Alzheimer's disease. While some of these disorders are, like Alzheimer's, chronic and incurable, others can be treated, reversed or cured completely. Many have nothing to do with the brain at all in relation to cause. Some of these disorders may also coexist with Alzheimer's, exaggerating symptoms.

There is always the need, in the case of memory loss and confusion, to have a complete diagnostic examination as soon as possible. This is true whether the confusion is mild or severe, whatever the person's age. The examination should include a thorough history and check-up, various blood tests, a neurological and psychological assessment and a psychiatric evaluation. The latter is generally done by a consultant in old age psychiatry. Old age psychiatrists work with people in hospital and community settings who suffer from functional and organic mental disorders.

Diagnosing Alzheimer's is a laborious process of elimination and exclusion. One visit to the doctor will not usually result in a diagnosis. Nor will one test.

Never feel guilty about seeking a second opinion. Diagnosis is difficult. The course of the disease process varies greatly from person to person, and there is always a degree of diagnostic uncertainty.

Members of Alzheimer's support groups can be particularly helpful in steering you towards sensitive doctors. Your district nurse may also be a good referral source. You'll want a GP you can talk to and trust because you'll probably be seeing a lot of each other. You might also appreciate one who is prepared to make home visits when necessary.

If you're uncomfortable with the doctor your loved one is currently seeing, enquire about doctors in your area who are specialists in geriatric medicine or neurology, experienced in diagnosing and treating dementing illnesses, or willing to make the appropriate referrals. Ask for information from your local Health Authority if needed; most have website information and can give you help in registering with a new GP as well as assistance in finding one if needed.

Evaluating a person for Alzheimer's is not a once-in-a-lifetime experience. Certain tests may need to be repeated annually or at more frequent intervals as the disease progresses, especially in younger people with Alzheimer's. Early symptoms of Alzheimer's disease are subtle, but if your loved one has Alzheimer's or some other type of chronic dementia, there will be a definite downhill progression. People with Alzheimer's do not get better.

For your own peace of mind and for the health of your loved one, never assume it's Alzheimer's until all the test results are in.

Historical Highlights

◄◄ *Actually, when we think back, Dad started to act depressed after his colostomy surgery in 1968. He felt he was not normal. But then there was more than just the depression. From that point on it seemed all downhill. There were other signs. He was about sixty-four.*

As carers, *we ourselves* are the single most important diagnostic tool in the search for truth about what's causing our loved one's confusion. Our reflections on the history of observed behaviour changes are invaluable to the doctor. Though most doctors will want to question a patient directly, people in the early stages of Alzheimer's can be masters in the fine art of 'cover-up'. Not a few doctors have been fooled by the perfectly normal behaviour and appearance of people with Alzheimer's in their surgery. You know things are different at home, but you may need some facts to prove it.

When attempting to reconstruct a medical and social history there are two key words to remember: *change* and *onset*.

What are the various changes you've noticed in your loved one's life over the past few weeks, months or years? When did you first notice these changes? Have they been gradual in onset, occurring over a period of time, or have they occurred suddenly?

The time frame for the appearance and progression of symptoms is an important clue for doctors to consider when making a diagnosis and deciding what tests to conduct. Before you go to the hospital or the GP's surgery, think through the following categories. You may even want to write down your answers and take them with you.

• *Affect and attitude:* Has your loved one been unusually anxious, agitated, depressed, apathetic or withdrawn? When did you first notice these changes? Have there been any major events associated with these changes, such as retirement, relocation, death of a close friend or relative, or surgery?

• *Behaviour.* What specific behaviour changes have you noticed? Have there been any differences in your loved one's daily routine? Have you noticed any marked personality changes, such as forgetfulness? If so, what exactly is forgotten? How frequently does forgetfulness occur?

• *Conversation.* Has your loved one experienced any language difficulties? Have there been any problems related to the ability to speak or remember words? Is one word substituted for another at the end of a sentence? Are phrases mixed up or confused? Has speech become slurred or garbled?

• *Decision making.* Have you noticed any changes in decision-making capabilities? Are there any errors in judgement? In relation to what, specifically? Is your loved one having difficulty driving? Is he/she able to do so safely? Has he or she ever wandered off and got lost?

• *Drugs.* List any medications being taken, both prescription and over-the-counter. Are medications being taken correctly?

• *Environment.* Are saucepans burned? Are there piles of unpaid bills? Is post stacked up? Is there evidence that your relative is neglecting nutritional needs?

• *Family and friends.* What have other people – friends, neighbours, co-workers – noticed about your loved one's behaviour?

• *Grooming and gait disturbances.* Is there any change in the person's ability to perform various activities of daily living related to personal grooming – bathing, dressing, toileting? Have there been any changes in the ability to walk or maintain their balance?

• *Habits.* What changes have you noticed in your loved one's normal habit patterns? Are there things that are simply too difficult to do now, such as balancing a cheque book, cooking, cleaning, reading, car repair, gardening? Are there any favourite hobbies that are no longer engaged in? Have you noticed any changes in the ability and desire to socialize with others?

• *Illnesses.* What specific physical symptoms is your loved one experiencing? Has there been any significant and recent weight loss or weight gain?

Is there a history of any of the following: metabolic disorders such as diabetes or thyroid disease, heart or lung abnormalities, strokes, dizziness, fainting spells, headaches, shaking, seizures? Is there any history of alcoholism?

Has your loved one fallen down or had any past or recent head injuries? Has there been exposure to any toxic chemicals in the workplace? Is there any history of blood transfusions? When and where were they done? Is there any history of Alzheimer's disease or undiagnosed memory loss in your loved one's family? Any familial nervous or mental disease?

As carers we need to be sure that no stone has been left unturned in the search for the cause of our loved one's confusion. The stones related to our loved one's history are the ones we need to turn over ourselves.

Maybe It's Not Alzheimer's

◄◄ *In the beginning we said to ourselves, 'Dad is just getting old.' Even his doctor said so and told us it was probably just hardening of the arteries to the brain. So we thought, well, he's getting old and he's getting senile.*

But his confusion wasn't just part of old age, we found out later. We finally took him to a doctor who listened to him, did a good examination and a bunch of tests, and who was willing to tell us more about what was going on.

A good place to start in the search for the truth about the cause of our loved one's confusion is with a general physical examination. This will involve more than taking a temperature, pulse and blood pressure.

Even if the primary dementia is caused by Alzheimer's, there may be associated chronic or acute problems. If these go undiagnosed and untreated, they can make the confusion caused by Alzheimer's worse. On the other hand, some of these conditions may themselves be the cause of the confusion.

Chronic and acute diseases and disabilities

Heart or lung-related diseases such as congestive heart failure, heart rhythm and valve disorders, pneumonia, and a variety of chronic obstructive lung disorders may contribute to mild or severe oxygen deprivation to the brain. This lack of oxygen, in turn, can cause acute episodes of confusion and can contribute to chronic dementia.

In some cases the culprit of confusion is a chronic cholesterol build-up that results in a narrowing of the arteries supplying blood to the brain. This is called coronary artery disease or atherosclerosis. Coronary artery disease (usually with accompanying hypertension) may, over a period of time, result in a series of small strokes or infarcts in the brain. These mini-strokes can cause an intermittent confusion that is frequently mistaken for Alzheimer's disease and often goes undetected unless the person experiences a massive stroke.

This mini-stroke phenomenon, more frequently seen in men, is a type of vascular dementia; it used to be called multi-infarct dementia. Vascular dementia is the second most common cause of irreversible dementia in older people.

Unlike Alzheimer's, vascular dementia often begins suddenly. Its downhill progression is variable, though often it is steplike in nature, with plateaus or periods of stability. There may be evidence of specific local or focal neurological impairments such as muscle weakness to an arm or leg, or slurred speech, as opposed to the more gradual and generalized global decline of Alzheimer's disease. By supplying the person's history, a carer may help the doctor to distinguish between Alzheimer's and vascular dementia.[2]

People can, and frequently do, suffer from vascular dementia in combination with Alzheimer's. Why is it important to know which problem is causing the person's confusion? Medical and/or surgical treatments can often reduce the likelihood of further stroke activity if the confusion is related to vascular disease rather than the Alzheimer's process. An accurate diagnosis can lead to improved health.

There are also other diseases that may produce progressive dementia-like symptoms. These diseases are also chronic and irreversible but treatments such as specific medications may differ, depending on the specific disease and its severity. Some of the most notable are: dementia with Lewy bodies, Huntington's chorea, fronto-temporal dementias such as Pick's disease, multiple sclerosis, amyotrophic lateral sclerosis, Parkinson's disease and Creutzfeldt-Jakob disease, an extremely rare brain disorder. An overview of each of these conditions and a more extensive discussion of vascular dementia is included in Appendix B.

Sensory impairments or disabilities may also be a factor in confusion. Occasionally when older people appear to be forgetful or confused, they are simply suffering from poor vision and/or hearing loss. Both conditions may be correctable with surgery or mechanical aids.

Deficiencies

The brain needs nutritious food to survive. A poorly nourished brain can contribute to confusion, forgetfulness, irritability and depression.

People – especially older people who live alone – can suffer from a number of conditions that are diet related. If older people forget to eat, or fail to eat enough of the right kinds of foods, they may wind up with nutritional deficiencies and even chronic malnutrition. Chronic alcoholism can also be a concern. Both conditions are associated with vitamin deficiencies, and some vitamin deficiencies contribute to dementia-like symptoms. If an older person is not drinking enough water, dehydration can also rapidly occur and contribute to lethargy and confusion and sometimes hallucinations. Food sensitivity can lead to confusion too.

Depression

Depression and manic depression are two other conditions that mimic Alzheimer's and should always be considered when there is memory loss.

Classically depressed people may appear passive, helpless, hopeless and confused. Behavioural and intellectual responses may be slower than normal. Manic depression may result in mood changes that swing between a state of excitement, or mania, and deep depression.

The onset of depression is usually more rapid than the onset of Alzheimer's and may be triggered by specific events such as the death of a spouse or the loss of a job. There are often accompanying physical signs such as fatigue, insomnia, and loss of weight and appetite. Social withdrawal and emotional withdrawal are common symptoms of both depression and Alzheimer's disease. A large-scale study of people over the age of sixty-five indicated that those who experienced symptoms of depression were more likely to eventually develop Alzheimer's.

Current research also indicates that depression frequently accompanies Alzheimer's, exaggerating the symptoms of dementia. Although Alzheimer's cannot be cured, depression will often respond to antidepressant medications.[3]

Drugs

One of the most commonly overlooked yet correctable causes of confusion in older people is drug toxicity. The effects of many medications extend far beyond the therapeutic purposes for which they were intended. Many have potentially harmful side effects that can include depression, disorientation and other dementia-like symptoms.

Drug toxicity can result from either a build-up of one specific medication or a combination of drugs that can produce toxic effects, usually over time. It's not unusual for an older person to be taking over a dozen different medications for various ailments, sometimes prescribed by several different physicians. Some of these drugs can neutralize other drugs when taken together. Or they can do the exact opposite and speed up the absorption of the second drug, often to an overdose level. All drugs, including those we may think of as innocuous over-the-counter pain relievers, cough suppressants and laxatives, have potential side effects.

Medications have a greater tendency to build up in the bodies of older people because of the decreased filtration rate in the kidneys. Poor circulation, slower general metabolism, constipation and a lower level of liver detoxification function contribute to drug toxicity as we age.

Medications can also adversely affect the proper absorption of vitamins, minerals and other nutrients. Overuse of some antacids, for example, can trigger thiamine deficiencies. Medications can also contribute to nutritional and electrolyte imbalances that, in turn, can create confusion. Even something as ordinary as a laxative, if taken indiscriminately, can upset fluid and electrolyte balances.

Older people sometimes consume alcohol in the form of wine or over-the-counter cough medicines or liquid vitamin supplements. Alcohol does not mix well with many medications. Confusion is a common side effect.

When we take our loved one to the hospital or to a doctor's surgery, we need to take their medications too, both prescription and over-the-counter, or at least have an accurate record of what they are taking and how long they've been taking it. Medication should definitely be considered as a contributing factor whenever dementia is suspected.

Don't Neglect the Lab Tests

⏮ *I think they did every test imaginable on my husband to make sure he wasn't suffering from something other than Alzheimer's. At forty-five, you want to make sure.*

No examination for Alzheimer's would be complete without blood analysis and other laboratory tests. All of them help to rule out other possible causes of dementia. While not every test will be used by every physician on every person showing symptoms of dementia, some of these certainly will be performed.

Blood tests

A full blood count (FBC) should be done to rule out the possibility of any underlying acute or chronic infectious process that can cause symptoms similar to Alzheimer's. The FBC can also detect other conditions such as blood cancers or anaemia. Low haemoglobin and haematocrit levels can contribute to confusion when there are not enough red blood cells carrying oxygen to the brain.

More specific blood chemistries can measure folic acid and vitamin B12 levels. Low vitamin B12 levels may be associated with pernicious anaemia. Symptoms include depression and irritability. Low B12 and folate levels also produce dementia-like symptoms.

Diabetes and other metabolic or endocrine disorders can contribute to marked irritability, personality changes and confusion. They can be detected by blood tests.

Abnormally high or low doses of thyroid hormone can trigger dementia-like symptoms and can be detected through various thyroid hormone level studies. Abnormally high levels of circulating calcium and sodium, and low sodium levels with accompanying electrolyte imbalances, can also trigger symptoms of dementia.

Poisoning with certain metals such as aluminium, manganese, lead or mercury has been implicated as a possible causative factor in dementia, as have pesticides, carbon monoxide and industrial pollutants. Blood levels can be tested for many of these.

In the nineteenth century, the number one cause of confusion was thought to be syphilis. While it is not generally a major cause of dementia today, a complete assessment for dementia may include a blood test for chronic venereal disease. Syphilis may still be prevalent in some areas today.

Acquired immune deficiency syndrome (AIDS) is another infectious process that can't be automatically ruled out. Dementia is a frequent complication of AIDS. Blood studies to detect the presence of the human immunodeficiency virus (HIV) may be done if the symptoms and health history indicate a need.

Urine tests

Urine testing can rule out an acute urinary tract infection that, in the elderly, may cause confusion; it can also increase confusion in people who have a diagnosed dementia. I worked as a research nurse on a multi-site nursing home project in the US, and my retrospective reviews of charts indicated that many nursing home residents with a diagnosis of Alzheimer's became increasingly confused and were often hospitalized as a result of urinary tract infections; the staff had initially attributed the confusion to behaviours associated with Alzheimer's rather than to an accompanying infection. High sugar and acetone readings in the urine can also indicate diabetes and the need for more extensive blood analysis. Urine and blood tests may also reveal evidence of medication overdose.

Spinal fluid tests

The spinal column is part of the central nervous system. The cerebral spinal fluid that courses through the spinal column also bathes the brain.

Spinal taps, or lumbar punctures (LPs), are recommended by some doctors as a diagnostic tool if there is reason to suspect they would help rule out an infectious process. In this procedure, a small amount of spinal fluid is withdrawn from the spinal column, then analyzed. Brain tumours, some blood-vessel diseases, and acute and chronic infectious processes such as meningitis and tuberculosis that cause confusion may be diagnosed through spinal taps.

The Mind Matters

When my mother was initially diagnosed with senile dementia of the Alzheimer's type, I went into the examining room with her when she saw the neurologist. I can still remember the 'conversation' my mother had with the young neurology resident.

'I just want to ask you a few questions,' the resident began.

'Okay,' my mother replied.

'What year is it?' he asked.

'1960,' she said.

'No, it's 1980,' he corrected her. 'What month is it?'

'May,' she said.

'No, it's December,' he said. 'What date is it now?'

'The first. Is that right?' my mother asked.

'No, it's the tenth,' he told her. 'What is the day of the week?'

'You're so clever, you tell me,' said Mum.

That concluded the mental-status exam.

What year is it now? What month is it? What date? What day of the week? For most of us, answers to these questions trip off our tongues without much thought. But for someone with a progressive memory loss like Alzheimer's, even the simplest questions can draw a blank.

◀◀ *The doctor never actually saw my father's bizarre behaviour. He wondered if it was my mother's imagination. Until he could see the problems for himself, he wouldn't believe her.*

The doctor finally took Dad into a room and asked him some questions.

Dad didn't know if he was married. He didn't know his religion. He didn't know who the president was. He didn't know the month or the day or the season.

The doctor finally realized my mother had been telling the truth.

A neurologist and/or the general practitioner may do a mental status or mini-mental status exam. The various tests that are part of the exam indicate the ability of different parts of the brain to function. The more complex questions can give clues to the cause and progression of the dementia.[4]

Mental status exams generally measure what is known as cognitive functioning. The word *cognition*, used extensively by health-care professionals when talking about the dementias, means 'the process or quality of knowing'. Cognition includes our ability to reason and remember, perceive and make judgements, conceive and imagine – all those mental activities that make us uniquely human, uniquely us.

Mental status exams may be repeated over time to better assess our loved one's level of functioning and rate of change. The questions used test a number of different areas:

• *Degree of orientation to time, place, person and object.* Do they know what day it is, where they are, who they are? Are they aware of current events? For example, do they know who the prime minister is? Do they know their phone number and their address? If shown familiar objects such as a pencil or a watch, can they name them?

• *Memory for remote and recent past.* Can they tell when and where they were born? Do they know the names of their parents? Can they repeat from memory a simple series of numbers or familiar objects five minutes after they are told what those numbers or objects are?

• *Mathematical skills.* Can they solve simple maths calculations? For example, can they count backwards from one hundred in multiples of three or four?

• *Abstract reasoning ability and judgement.* Do they know the meaning of simple proverbs such as 'A bird in the hand is worth two in the bush'? If they were told the cooker was on fire in their kitchen, what would they do? Is their response logical?

• *Reading, writing and symbolic drawing skills.* Are they able to read? Do they understand what they are reading? Are they able to construct a sentence or a paragraph? Can they copy a simple design such as two overlapping triangles or rectangles? Can they draw the face of a clock and pencil in the appropriate numbers in the right places?

We often take our minds for granted. The mental status exam reminds us of how much they really do matter and of how they can be adversely affected by a disease such as Alzheimer's.

Having Your Head Examined

We're all familiar with the phrase 'You ought to have your head examined.' This, in fact, may be just what the doctor orders for a confused person who may be suffering from Alzheimer's disease. When my mother began having symptoms of memory loss, the last thing she wanted to do was to go to a doctor. 'I don't trust them,' she'd say when my father and I encouraged her to visit a nearby clinic.

I finally made an appointment with the practice nurse in our small town. I thought the fact that she was a woman might help make my mother feel more at ease, and I thought the small office would seem less imposing than a big hospital.

I was wrong on both counts.

My mother reluctantly agreed to the appointment, but we hadn't been in the waiting room more than five minutes when she headed out of the door at top speed. 'I'm all right,' she insisted. 'All right.'

One day, after several more episodes like this, I got a call at work from the local supermarket. Mum had been seen in town making her usual morning rounds from post office to coffee shop to local food store. The store manager had noticed my mother seemed more confused than usual. 'The side of her mouth is drooping a bit,' he said. 'She's unsteady on her feet, but she keeps insisting she's okay and won't let me call an ambulance.'

I got in my car and drove the eight miles home in about five minutes. There was my mother coming out of the bank, leaning to the left. I knew the signs. She looked as if she'd had a small stroke.

'Get in the car, Mum,' I said.

'No.'

'Mum, please get in the car.'

'No,' she insisted.

Thankfully, my mother was small. I got out and manoeuvred her into the car, fastened her seat belt, and drove to the hospital. She protested all the way but calmed down as we neared the emergency entrance.

When we got there, I was able to speak to a doctor I knew. He seized the opportunity to admit her and then give her a brain or CT scan. A short time later, she was officially diagnosed as having Alzheimer's. There was no evidence on the scan of any past stroke activity.

Other carers have shared their initial experience with the diagnostic process.

⏮ *My wife had been going to one hospital for her eyes. Laser treatments. And one day her doctor said, 'You know, it wouldn't hurt your wife to have an MRI scan done.' I asked why.*

He said, 'Well, in talking to her there are times when she doesn't answer me.'

I said to him, 'I know that. I thought she was just ignoring me.'

'No,' he said. 'It's much more than that.'

A thorough neurological examination for mental impairment may include an EEG, CT or MRI scan either early in the investigative process or after more simple tests have been done without a diagnosis being made.[5]

The EEG, or electroencephalogram, measures electrical activity in the brain. It involves attaching tiny wires called electrodes to the side of the head with a paste-like substance. The brain waves of people with Alzheimer's may appear perfectly normal, or they may show abnormally slow electrical activity. EEGs can help identify other causes of dementia with symptoms that mimic Alzheimer's such as delirium and various seizure disorders, like epilepsy, that may have gone undiagnosed or been misdiagnosed in the past.

A CT scan, or computed axial tomography, is a computer-drawn X-ray of the brain itself. Normally we all experience a certain degree of brain atrophy or shrinkage and brain-weight loss as we get older, due to a decreased number of living brain cells. Alzheimer's disease speeds up the process of cellular shrinkage and cellular death significantly. CT scans can measure brain atrophy by indicating space between the skull and the brain related to widespread loss of nerve tissue in the cerebral cortex, or outer covering of the brain. A diagnosis of mild to severe atrophy can be made, depending on the size of the space. Usually, but not always, the greater the degree of dementia, the greater the atrophy. Atrophy is greatest in the frontal, temporal and parietal regions of the cortex.

Inner spaces of the brain, or ventricles, where cerebrospinal fluid normally circulates, also increase in size as brain substance decays and is replaced by more fluid. Some research has indicated cerebral atrophy and ventricular enlargement to be greater in persons with suspected dementia of the Alzheimer's type compared to persons with vascular dementias, though ventricular size and degree of Alzheimer's dementia do not appear closely related.

Magnetic resonance imaging, known as MRI or NMR, is a more recently developed head-examining technique. MRI provides a more detailed picture of the brain than a CT scan, and may be ordered if CT scan results are judged insufficient to make a diagnosis.

Unfortunately, the CT scan or MRI alone can't provide an absolute diagnosis of Alzheimer's disease. Brain shrinkage is not always apparent. In any case, the only absolute proof is found through brain post-mortem (autopsy) following death. But what these tests *can* do, in conjunction with other tests, is eliminate other possible causes of dementia. Scans can detect brain tumours, cysts, blood clots or subdural haematomas that may have resulted from falls or blows to the head; normal-pressure hydrocephalus, or an excess of fluid on the brain; and the stroke activity of vascular dementia.

Pick's disease, a dementia that produces lesser degrees of memory loss than Alzheimer's but greater degrees of socially and sexually inappropriate behaviour, may also be detected. It is evidenced by severe atrophy in the area of the temporal cortex of the brain. Again, this diagnosis is not conclusive apart from brain post-mortem.

In addition to EEGs and CT and MRI scans, PET (positron emission tomography) procedures, which complement rather than replace the more common types of structural imaging methods, are sometimes done in research facilities.

In the PET procedure, radioactive glucose is injected into the brain and studies are done to determine what areas of the brain are able to metabolize the glucose. If someone suffers from Alzheimer's, it is anticipated that there will be certain 'dead' areas in the brain, most notably in the temporal and parietal lobes, where no metabolism will take place.

An even more recent diagnostic tool is called SPECT (single photon emission computed tomography). This is a procedure researchers hope will help separate treatable types of dementia from irreversible types such as Alzheimer's.

EEGs, CT and MRI scans, and PET and SPECT procedures are not painful, but they may be frightening to a person who is confused to begin with. They are usually done in busy hospitals on stretchers or tables that are cold, hard and uncomfortable. If a person fails to relax or is moving around, it may be difficult to get accurate test results. Mild sedation may be ordered prior to the test.

Reassurance, going with your loved one to the examination area (something you may have to insist on), and appealing to your loved one's sense of humour may all be necessary. One carer told his wife that having a CT scan was like going to the beauty parlour. When she arrived at the hospital, she was delighted. The bowl-shaped CT scanner looked like a giant hair dryer. Once her head was in place, she promptly fell asleep.

If a person's symptoms are of recent onset, one or more of the foregoing procedures may be done. If symptoms have advanced and progressed for several years, they may not be. But they are all options to consider when you and your relative's doctor are searching for the truth.

Chapter Three

Facing the Facts

Every day at 11:00 a.m. the taxi pulls up in front of the terraced house on Victoria Road. The driver toots, turns off the engine, lights a cigarette and waits for Ralph Murphy, who will soon appear with an umbrella in one hand, a shopping bag in the other, and an overcoat thrown over his shoulder. Ralph will suddenly disappear again because he's forgotten to feed the cat, check the rings on the cooker or turn out the lights. But he's seventy-five and entitled to a little memory lapse, thinks the taxi driver.

'Hi ya, Jack.'

'Hi ya, Mr Murphy. The usual, right?'

'Right, Jack. Same time. Same station. Every day. You know me. Can't keep a good man down.'

The taxi inches its way along and finally stops in front of a two-storey brick building surrounded by azaleas. The sign on the door reads Riverview Manor Convalescent Home.

'See you at 2:30,' says Ralph Murphy, handing Jack a ten-pound note.

'I'll be here,' says the driver. 'Say hello to Mrs Murphy for me.'

'Will do, Jack. Will do.'

Inside, he calls out, 'Harriet, love, I'm here. It's your Ralph.'

Harriet Murphy doesn't turn to acknowledge her husband. Instead, she's looking out of her window, pointing with her finger in the general direction of the car park across the street.

'What are you looking at, Honey?'

Harriet doesn't respond. She just continues to point.

'It's about time for dinner. Are you ready, Honey?' asks Ralph.

'Hungry,' says Harriet, looking at her husband for the first time.

'That's my girl.'

Ralph lays his coat and umbrella on the bed, puts his shopping bag in Harriet's lap, grips the handles of her wheelchair, and propels it out of the door. They head for the dining room of the nursing home where one tray waits for Harriet and another waits for him, courtesy of the management. Ralph feeds Harriet her dinner and then eats his own, as he has every day for the past four years.

After dinner they go out onto the patio and look at the birds around the bird table, and Ralph talks to Harriet. He tells her stories about the children and grandchildren and great-grandchildren, and they look at all the pictures he keeps in the shopping bag.

Then Ralph wheels Harriet back to her room. He kisses her goodbye, tells her he loves her, goes out to the desk, jokes with the nurses for a few minutes, heads for the lobby, gets into his waiting taxi and leaves.

'How'd it go today, Mr Murphy?' asks Jack.

'Not so good, not so good.'

Jack doesn't say anything more. He knows that today Ralph Murphy just wants to sit back and remember.

It's been a long time since that day in June. Over fifteen years. But Ralph still remembers it as though it were yesterday. You don't forget a thing like that. It's not every day your wife accuses you of being a rapist.

They'd stopped at a motorway service station on their way up to Scotland.

Ralph had got out to get them a couple of sandwiches and some coffee. When he came back to the car, there they were: Harriet, two policemen and a crowd of onlookers.

Before he could open his car door, the questions started.

'Are you the man who claims to be Ralph Murphy?'

'I am Ralph Murphy,' he said. 'What's the matter?'

'This woman claims you kidnapped her, raped her and are holding her against her will.'

At that point Ralph started laughing.

'What's so funny?'

'She's my wife,' Ralph repeated. 'My wife. She gets very confused sometimes. Haven't you talked to her?'

'Yes, we did,' said the policeman. 'And you're right. She did seem confused. She told us it was 1931 and a few other things that didn't make much sense. I guess maybe you're right. You act like you're her husband, but you're still going to have to prove it. Is there someone we can call?'

'My son. In Scotland. That's where we were heading.'

So Ralph gave the police the number and they made the call. His son verified that Ralph was indeed his father, that Harriet was his mother and that, yes, she had been having some memory problems.

'If you've got any more stops to make, Mr Murphy,' said the policeman, 'you might want to cancel your trip. Either that or don't let your wife out of your sight. We believed you. The next time you might not be so lucky.'

The next morning, Ralph and Harriet Murphy headed back to Dorset.

The following week, Ralph made an appointment at the health centre. When he came out of the doctor's surgery two weeks later with a tentative diagnosis of Alzheimer's disease, he suspected there'd be no more trips to Scotland. He couldn't deny the decline any longer.

The next few years were hell on earth for him. Harriet's suspicions grew worse. She continued accusing him of molesting her. 'I don't know you. Get out!' she'd scream at him if he tried to come into their bedroom.

He tried to tell Harriet she had an illness when she asked, as she often did, what was wrong with her. 'You have an illness of your mind,' he'd say. Then she'd get upset and accuse him of being crazy.

Then there was the night she ran away. Luckily he was a light sleeper. He got up and stumbled downstairs when he realized she was gone. He headed for the bridge. And sure enough, there was Harriet getting ready to jump off.

This time Ralph was grateful to see the police who were patrolling the area. They helped him get her into the car and take her home.

'You know, you're going to need some help with her,' one of the policemen said.

'I know,' he said. 'I know.'

Three weeks later, Harriet was admitted to Riverview Manor. She hated the place at first. She accused the nurses, the cleaners, even the nursing home administrator of molesting her, of holding her against her will. And Ralph knew she talked to them about him. What a terrible person he'd been to her. How unfeeling he was for 'dumping her' like this.

But Harriet was safe. She was clean, dry and fed. She was well taken care of. For that, he was grateful.

'Same time tomorrow, Mr Murphy?' asks the driver, pulling up in front of the terraced house.

'Same time, same station. Thanks, Jack.'

Ralph Murphy gets out of the taxi, pays the driver, waves and starts up the steps. When he reaches the top step he pauses, turns around and doubles back to the waiting taxi. He's forgotten his overcoat.

Blowing Away the Myths

'In short, I believe that the major diseases of human beings have become approachable biological puzzles, ultimately solvable... Strokes and senile dementia, and cancer, and arthritis are not natural aspects of the human condition, and we ought to rid ourselves of such impediments as quickly as we can,' wrote Dr Lewis Thomas in *The Medusa and the Snail*.[1] In addition to chronic and dementing diseases, another impediment we need to rid ourselves of is myths.

In relation to dementia in general and Alzheimer's in particular, myths abound. There's a lot of fiction mixed in with the facts largely arising out of fear and/or lack of knowledge.

Myth number 1: All old people get senile

All confused people age, but not all people who age become confused. Chronology is not synonymous with confusion.

In actual fact, only about 5 per cent of all people between the ages of sixty-five and seventy are moderately to severely impaired intellectually due to dementia. That leaves 95 per cent of people in this age bracket with minds that, intellectually speaking, function very well indeed, though there is a significant increase in Alzheimer's after the age of eighty.

Any sign of forgetfulness in our loved ones or even ourselves should not trigger a panic attack. Just because you forgot where you put your car keys, missed an appointment with your dentist, or can't remember where you stored last summer's picnic supplies does not mean you're in the early stages of Alzheimer's. Isolated instances of forgetfulness may simply be related to information overload or the natural memory loss we all experience from time to time.

Part One: Something Has Gone Wrong

As we grow up we grow old, and our brains are included in this ageing process. Any one of us, if we live into our seventies, eighties or nineties, will undoubtedly experience a small degree of forgetfulness. That's because the senile plaques and neurofibrillary tangles that are so characteristic of Alzheimer's are also present in normal ageing brains. But, unlike the plaques and tangles of Alzheimer's, they are scattered throughout the brain and are fewer in number. Although these changes in the brain can contribute to occasional memory lapses, especially when we're under stress, they don't result in full-blown dementia for everyone.

Myth number 2: If you keep your mind active and read more books, you definitely won't get Alzheimer's

Alzheimer's is no respecter of persons. It knows no social, sexual, ethnic, occupational or educational boundaries. There are no current indications that Alzheimer's disease or any of the other incurable dementias can absolutely be prevented or staved off by keeping your mind and body active in your youth or later years. There have been recent studies done, however, on correlations between an active lifestyle in general and possible lower risks for dementia, with regular midlife exercise being a possible protective factor. Clearly that could help reduce the risk from certain types of dementia such as vascular dementia, though the relationship between exercise and dementia of the Alzheimer's type is less clear.

Myth number 3: Alzheimer's disease is contagious

Alzheimer's is *not* contagious. You can't catch it as you can AIDS or the flu. It's not bloodborne or airborne; it is related to a specific disease process. There has been some research conducted on a virus as a possible causative factor but at present the findings indicate this is unlikely. (See Appendix C for more information.)

Myth number 4: There are many treatments for Alzheimer's disease

To date, there are some recommended medications used to treat symptoms associated with Alzheimer's disease, but there is no definitive treatment. There are, however, many false prophets in the world eager to take our hard-earned money. They advocate any number of cures and correctives and sometimes even try to pinpoint a specific cause for Alzheimer's. Bogus remedies range from massive doses of megavitamins to herbal therapies and more. When we see our loved one deteriorating before our eyes, it's only natural to want to grasp at any available straw if there's even a remote possibility it may help alleviate some of the symptoms of Alzheimer's and slow the disease process. But it's also natural and in our best interests to ask questions before investing our money in something that, in the long run, could make our loved one's condition worse. The claims of alternative treatments should be examined cautiously.

When in doubt about an advertised home-remedy or an expensive treatment offered in some out-of-the-way place, the best thing to do is nothing – until you have consulted your GP or called or written to the Alzheimer's Society (see Appendix D) and requested information. The Society can also give you information about legitimate experimental drug trials being conducted with Alzheimer's sufferers. There are a number in progress. Additional information about some of the current medications used to treat Alzheimer's and promising research is included in Appendix C.

Myth number 5: The confusion could easily be cleared up if the blood flowed better. I've heard there are pills you can take that dilate the blood vessels

Some drugs, called *vasodilators*, increase the diameter of the blood vessels in the brain. Alzheimer's, however, is not a vascular disease, and many physicians believe that vasodilators can in fact be harmful to elderly people with Alzheimer's-type dementia. Vasodilators also dilate peripheral blood vessels in the arms and legs and can actually reduce the pressure available for adequate cerebral blood flow. Decreased blood pressure, such as that which frequently occurs when a person suddenly stands up, can result in lightheadedness and falls, especially in people with Alzheimer's who have difficulty maintaining balance and coordination. If used at all, vasodilators should be taken with caution and carefully evaluated by both doctor and carer.

The Aluminium Question

Although it has been known for some time that higher-than-normal concentrations of aluminium salts have been found in the brain cells of people who suffered from Alzheimer's and other dementias, most researchers believed that excess aluminium was the result, not the cause, of the disease. However, there is a growing amount of circumstantial evidence linking aluminium with Alzheimer's disease in some way, and research continues.

Beware, however, of websites promoting do-it-yourself oral chelation therapy to 'cure' Alzheimer's by ridding the body of excess aluminium through a detoxifying process. The only safe use of this and related treatments is under close medical supervision and, to date, most of this treatment has been in the context of clinical trials. The Alzheimer's Society has stated that the research findings do not at this time indicate any causal relationship between aluminium and Alzheimer's disease.

The following are reasons for some concern, however, and indicate the need for further research:

• Aluminium is one of the few substances known to cause brain tangles and memory loss when injected into certain animals, though the tangles do appear to differ in structure and composition from those that occur in people.

• Aluminium was identified as the cause of 'dialysis dementia', suffered by some patients undergoing dialysis for kidney disease. This condition was reversed by removing aluminium from the dialysis fluid.

• Some earlier research in the UK suggests that rates of Alzheimer's disease were approximately one and a half times more frequent in districts with higher levels of aluminium in the water, compared with those in which it was low or absent;

the methodology and findings of some of the studies have been questioned.

Aluminium is one of the most common metals in our environment. We are daily exposed to its chemical forms in the food we eat, the water, tea and coffee we drink, the medications we take, and even some deodorants we use. Some people also experience occupational exposure to dust containing aluminium or aluminium compounds.

None of this is proof that aluminium contributes to the degenerative changes that cause Alzheimer's disease. However, it may be that some people are more at risk because of genetic or other factors and would benefit from a reduction of their intake of aluminium. For the present, you may feel that it is prudent to avoid foods containing aluminium additives and to use non-aluminium pans and utensils, particularly for cooking acidic foods which are known to leach more aluminium from the pan.

Further research is needed before any definite conclusions can be drawn. It is helpful to remember that even if a clear link is found with Alzheimer's, the risk from any past or present exposure to aluminium is still small. Iron, zinc and mercury are three other elements being studied by researchers.[2]

At present, there is not a vast array of treatments or any cure for Alzheimer's disease, but different medications are being tested and used for symptom control. There is also hope. Alzheimer's is not a normal process of ageing. It is a disease, a deviation from the norm. And, as we've learned through experience over the years, diseases *are* solvable biological puzzles that may one day reveal to us the reasons for their existence.

Don't Deny the Decline

◄◄ *My aunt became very frustrated. She knew there was something desperately wrong with her, and she would sit in her chair and whimper a lot. She always had this sad, sad look. And she thought – and we thought – she was losing her mind.*

⏮ *There were other things, as I look back, that I should have noticed about my wife. In November of 1976 she wanted to have our wills made out. She kept insisting. I wonder if she knew something then I didn't know or even suspect?*

⏮ *'What's the use?' I remember my husband saying to me when he first started to lose his memory. 'What's the point of living?'*

People in the early stages of Alzheimer's disease need all the support they can get from family, friends, relatives and the community. They need to be assured they aren't going crazy, that life is not over for them, that they are still loved and accepted.

Denial is a very common reaction to the diagnosis of Alzheimer's and to the initial symptoms of memory loss, even before a diagnosis is made. We may deny initial symptoms because our loved one's behaviour doesn't fit our expectations of a disease. Most people are used to equating illness with observable signs. People with Alzheimer's usually look healthy and alert. They may, in fact, have considerably more energy than we do. Instead of blaming a disease, we attribute their confusion to the myth of senility, or to various changes that occur in mid-to-late life.

⏮ *I didn't realize there was anything wrong with my husband for a very long time. He was always so healthy and still is, even though he's been diagnosed with Alzheimer's for over four years.*

In the beginning I just thought his memory problems were part of his ageing, and I guess I thought that if your mind was slipping badly your body should be falling apart too. His wasn't.

⏮ *My mother was always a little eccentric and a bit of a loner. She just seemed to get more eccentric as the years progressed. She withdrew from life more and more after she retired. But she looked so healthy we didn't worry about it.*

⏮ *Actually we thought Mum was going through menopause. She seemed to have all the signs and symptoms, though they were a bit exaggerated.*

We may deny out of shame or embarrassment. In past generations, families with relatives who were mentally ill or mentally handicapped kept them 'in the cupboard', so to speak. They never talked about them outside the immediate family. And, in some cases, people *literally* kept their relatives in the cupboard.

For some families there's still a stigma attached to mental illness and mental handicap. This stigma can carry over into the way we feel about a loved one with dementia.

We may also think people outside our immediate family won't understand our loved one's bizarre behaviour and will judge us. We're sure they're saying, 'There's Harry again, acting strange. Why doesn't Virginia *do* something?'

So, embarrassed by our friend's or loved one's behaviour, we try to protect everyone involved from potentially awkward or distressing situations.

⏮ *In the beginning we didn't know what was happening to Dad. When he started acting strange in front of other people, we were embarrassed. We tried to cover it up because of our embarrassment. Actually we ourselves were immature.*

⏮ *My wife would make a fool of herself in restaurants. She'd say suggestive things to the waiters and waitresses. One time she even pinched a waiter on the rear. I was embarrassed to death and apologized for her behaviour. Then, finally, I stopped taking her out altogether.*

We may deny because the truth is too painful to accept.

⏮ *My daughter will sit next to her mother for hours at a time now and her mother won't speak to her, won't recognize her. I know it's hard on her. Awfully hard.*

My daughter didn't want to accept her mother's sickness

*in the first place. The doctor told her, 'You've got to start
accepting it. You've got to tell your children what's going
on. It's not going to get better.'*

  And the doctor was right. It didn't.

There's also a natural tendency for us to want to preserve the lives
and livelihoods of our loved ones for as long as possible.

◀◀ *I wrote my husband's cover letters for him when he was
applying for jobs. I knew it was stupid. He wouldn't have been
able to do any of those jobs anyway. But I didn't want to see
him give up. It was denial, I guess. Either that or blind faith.*

◀◀ *There was a lot of denial on my part. I didn't want things
to end. I didn't want him not to be able to drive any more. His
self-esteem was so shaken anyway that I just wanted him to do
what he could for as long as possible... So I let him drive, even
when I knew he wasn't safe on the road. And I prayed a lot.*

It's very easy for us as carers to deny the truth because our loved ones
deny it as well. They can make tremendous efforts to compensate for
their failing faculties.

◀◀ *I'm sure my husband had Alzheimer's for several years
before he was diagnosed. But he was always so good at
concealing his memory loss. He joked about it a lot, about how
when he got older he just had so many more things to think
about that it was easy to have more things to forget. I thought
that made sense.*

Sometimes the health professionals don't help our situation and, at
times, they can even make it worse. Even doctors aren't immune to
the myth of senility.

◀◀ *For three years my husband told the doctors he was
having trouble with his memory. For three years the doctors
kept telling him, 'Everybody does when they get to a certain
age.'*

*Finally things got so bad my husband couldn't perform
his job. They finally started to listen.*

In the case of Alzheimer's, we might sometimes feel as though we'd
rather not know. But ignorance is not really bliss. To be forewarned
is to be forearmed. There are six good reasons why, sooner or later,
we have to stop denying.

Six Reasons to Face the Facts

1. Information drives away fear

Early recognition of Alzheimer's disease can help us deal with our
own fears more realistically. One reason Alzheimer's is so frightening
is that it makes us feel out of control. We can't prevent it, arrest it or
stop it. One of the best ways to allay this fear is through knowledge
and understanding of the disease itself. There are many reputable
sources from which we can get reliable information. The more
information we have to draw from, the better able we'll be to cope
with this devastating disease.

One of the best sources of reliable information is the Alzheimer's
Society. The Alzheimer's Society (formerly the Alzheimer's Disease
Society) was founded in 1979, and many regional branches have
been formed as well as relatives' support groups in many parts of
Britain. There are Alzheimer's societies or associations in many
countries. Most have websites with extensive information about all
aspects of Alzheimer's and printable resource materials for carers.
The Alzheimer's Society does all of the following:

• It supports research into the causes and possible cures for
Alzheimer's disease and other forms of dementia.

• It helps organize carer support groups to assist, encourage and
educate carers.

• It sponsors educational programmes and provides written
and audio-visual information on Alzheimer's disease and related
disorders for both professional and nonprofessional carers.

• It advocates for carers and people with Alzheimer's disease in areas of legislation – locally, nationally and internationally.

The earlier we are aware of information and available resources, the less likely we are to be faced with a full-blown crisis later, when management problems become increasingly difficult and we need outside help.[3]

2. Our loved ones must be kept safe
Denial can become dangerous – especially for the loved one living alone, as many people do in the early stages of Alzheimer's.

If our loved one is in danger of falling, of setting the house on fire because of forgetfulness, or of wandering off and getting lost, the time has come to actively intervene, whether we want to or not. Independence is not something that can be preserved indefinitely for someone with Alzheimer's.

This recognition of danger may not mean suddenly uprooting loved ones and moving them in with us, but it will mean providing for their safety in practical ways, such as hiring home-care workers or a live-in companion.

3. Our loved ones may benefit from ongoing research
The majority of medications currently prescribed for Alzheimer's sufferers were first used in clinical trials and many carers also credit experimental drug trials with alleviating some of the symptoms of the disease for their relatives. Drug trials are being conducted all over the world at various hospitals and research centres. The earlier the diagnosis, the greater the chance an Alzheimer's sufferer will qualify for a programme should he or she wish to do so. Local or regional support groups or chapters can help identify various locations where studies are going on. The Alzheimer's Society can also provide information. (See also Appendices C and D.)

4. The entire family should play a role in caring
Alzheimer's disease is a family affair. In most instances, spouses,

siblings, children, grandchildren, great-grandchildren and an assortment of in-laws are involved. All have roles and responsibilities when it comes to caring, and open communication early in the course of the disease is important to ensure that the burden of caring is shared.

5. Financial arrangements must be made
Alzheimer's not only bankrupts the mind; it can also take its toll on family finances and savings accounts. There are many hidden costs involved in caring at home and the carer's potential for earning is obviously affected. Residential care, nursing home care and home care can all be expensive so it is best to explore all the options. Personal care provision provided in homes through Social Services is a means tested service based on income and savings to determine what costs, if any, are the responsibility of the person receiving care. The prospects of long-term care – with costs that continue to rise – can create panic. Long-term care sponsored by the National Health Service, for example, is not entirely free across the UK, though there are exceptions. In England, Wales and Northern Ireland, certain criteria must be met to qualify for free care. It is important to be aware of the benefits available to carers and those with Alzheimer's, and to claim those to which you are entitled.

The best advice for carers is to become aware of legalities governing estates and the care of older people in varying situations. Various avenues for legal advice include the Citizens Advice Bureau, the Law Centre, a private solicitor or the Court of Protection. At the earliest possible stage, carers need to consider obtaining an Enduring Power of Attorney enabling them to take charge of their loved one's affairs when it becomes necessary to do so. It is also worth knowing that sufferers from dementia should be exempt from paying Council Tax.[4]

The Alzheimer's Society has published information sheets on various aspects of legal and financial arrangements and can also offer advice relevant to specific situations.

6. The future must be planned

An early diagnosis of Alzheimer's can give both you and your loved one time to think together about what you would do if you had a future with many long years ahead of you. Then, think about living out the future *now*. For example, you may want to take early retirement or go on that trip you've been putting off.

Memory loss in the early stages of Alzheimer's does not mean people are incapable of making any rational decisions. On the contrary, they need to be involved in planning their own future to as great a degree as possible. This may even include the difficult decision of whether or not they want to be resuscitated should they have a cardiac or respiratory arrest in the later stages of their illness.

Alzheimer's is a fatal disease. It's been called a terminal illness that results in a slow death of the mind. As with any terminal illness, it is a natural initial reaction to deny. Our denial of Alzheimer's disease acts as a cushion. It softens the blow to protect us early on from the emotional pain and distress we might otherwise not be able to handle. Yet to finally admit that our loved ones are experiencing more than 'just a little memory loss' can be a relief – for them and for us.

One carer I interviewed told me about an experience her young son had. They were at a family picnic on a beach near a group of people who suffered from mild to severe mental and physical disabilities.

◄◄ *'A lot of the other children seemed afraid of them,' said the carer. 'Their behaviour was a bit different, and many of the children seemed to be intentionally avoiding them. They'd back away. But not my son. He said, "Look, Mummy. There are some sick people from the hospital."*

'My son certainly wasn't afraid of them. He walked right up to their group, reached out, shook some of their hands and introduced himself. I think it had a lot to do with him spending so much time with his grandmother who has Alzheimer's. He's used to being around people whose behaviour is different.'

We can learn a lot from this young child. As carers we need to have the courage to walk up to the disease, look it squarely in the eye, and shake it by the hand. We need to say, 'I am not afraid of you, and I'm not going to deny your existence.' And we need to say to our loved one, 'I love you. I'm not ashamed of your behaviour. We'll fight this disease together.' It's this kind of realistic and healthy attitude that can carry us beyond the inevitable denial and move us into acceptance.

Chapter Four

What's Happening Upstairs?

Well, here they were again. It was 4:00 p.m. on a Friday afternoon and they were headed for the café. Precisely at 3:00 p.m., Anna had started pacing up and down, up and down, in the kitchen at home, repeating the same old question, 'When are we going? When are we going? When are we going to go?' The same question she'd asked nearly every afternoon for the past six months.

Sam couldn't understand it.

His daughter had tried to explain it to him. 'It's part of her disease, Dad. She can't help it. People with Alzheimer's often repeat themselves, over and over again.'

Damnedest disease he'd ever seen. Why couldn't she have got sugar diabetes or broken her hip? That you could live with. But no, Anna had to go and get senile.

Funny thing about it was she'd always been so clever. Always had her head in a book. Did the taxes. Kept the cheque book. Paid the bills.

Now Sam had to do all those things. All those things he didn't like. He'd never had a head for figures. Anna was the brains of the outfit.

He certainly didn't expect retirement to be like this. They were supposed to be able to relax and enjoy life after forty years of working in the factory. Both of them. Forty years apiece. They'd retired at the same time, five years ago. They'd planned to move to Canada.

Canada! Ha! Anna couldn't even go around the block without getting lost. Imagine what would happen if they went to Canada! She'd probably wind up in some remote place with Sam searching for her. They'd both die of exposure.

She'd forgotten how to cook, too. Anna had always been such a good cook. Nothing fancy – just your basic meat and potatoes. But good meat and good potatoes. And always ready when Sam was hungry. They used to love to eat. After work, Anna would cook a big meal, then maybe they'd watch the news on TV, go over to their daughter's house and spend some time with the grandchildren. That is, until their daughter's husband got transferred to Germany. That put an end to that.

Now Sam and Anna didn't eat at home much any more except when Sam did the cooking, and Sam hated to cook. Never could figure out how to poach an egg just right or even make a good cup of coffee. And he did like his poached eggs and coffee.

Cooking, cleaning, paying the bills. All these things Sam had to do now, if he wanted them done at all. Too much, he thought. Too much.

'When we gonna get there? When we gonna get there?'

Anna snapped Sam out of his musings as the car pulled up at the café, seven miles from home.

'We're here, Hon, we're here.'

'Good. Let's eat,' said Anna.

Sam opened his door, went around the car, and helped Anna out. She brushed off his hand as if it were a fly and ran up the steps of the café.

'Hi, Sam. Hi, Anna. Want a menu?' asked Bill, the owner.

'No. You know we don't need one,' Sam said as they sat down in the booths by the row of windows.

'Menu. Menu. Menu,' said Anna.

'Oh, all right. Give us a menu. She can look. I'll order.'

'Looks like she's been putting on some weight again. You too. Guess that's good, huh, Sam?' said Bill.

'Yeah,' said Sam. 'Anna never eats much when we're home. Guess she doesn't like my cooking. Guess that's why you're still in business, because of people like us.'

'So what'll it be today?'

'The usual. Two egg and chips. Two coffees.'

'No,' said Anna, peering over her menu and glaring at her husband. 'No. No. No.'

'Oh, I almost forgot,' said Sam. 'And two big pieces of apple pie.' Anna smiled.

'Give me the menu, Anna,' said Sam.

'No. No. No. No.'

'That's all right, Sam. She can keep it.'

'Thanks, Bill. Give her something to look at while we're waiting. Give her something to read. She always did like to read. I wonder what went wrong? What went wrong?'

'My mind is all mixed up. Like this,' my mother once said to me, holding up a tangled purple strand of wool she was attempting to crochet into one of her famous afghans.

Mixed up. Tangled. Like a skein of wool that's slowly being unravelled by a precocious kitten. That's a fairly accurate picture of someone experiencing symptoms of Alzheimer's disease.

Alzheimer's is not a normal result of ageing. It's related to a specific disease process. Very distinct pathological changes take place in the brain. Under a microscope some of these changes *do* resemble a tangled skein of wool.

When someone we love is 'all mixed up' because of a confusion-causing disease like Alzheimer's, it's important to have as much information as possible to better understand the disease process.

But to understand what goes wrong, we first need to take a look at what's normal. How are our brains supposed to work? How are they structured? Just what *does* go on inside our heads, anyway?

The brain is, quite literally, the headquarters for the rest of the body. It's the main office, the control tower, the central meeting place for a vast network of nerves that control all our conscious activity and affect our unconscious actions as well.

The brain isn't much to look at. On the surface it rather resembles a three-pound walnut. But beneath the grey and convoluted exterior of the brain is housed a complex information storage and retrieval system that is responsible for memory, thoughts, language, behaviour and emotions.

The brain consists of three main parts: the cerebrum, or large brain; the cerebellum, or small brain; and the brain stem.

The *cerebrum* fills nearly the entire brain cavity and consists of two cerebral hemispheres covered by a grey outer covering called the *cerebral cortex*. This 'grey matter' is associated with our higher mental functions.

The *cerebellum*, located at the back of the brain cavity and below the cerebrum, is responsible for balance and coordinates muscular activity.

The *brain stem* connects the brain to the spinal column and controls the vital functions of breathing and circulation.

To illustrate how a normal brain works, and to better understand what goes wrong when a person becomes afflicted with Alzheimer's, let's look at one specific activity our brains are engaged in every day: making decisions.

The brain, like the rest of our organs, is made up of billions of microscopic cells. In the brain these cells are called *neurons*. Each neuron is composed of a cell body or *soma*, short, branching shoots called *dendrites*, and a long, threadlike structure called an *axon*. Dendrites from one cell conduct electrical stimulation received from other cells; the axon transmits or carries nerve signals away from the cell or soma. At the end of axon terminals are spaces or junctions known as *synapses*.

Let's say we decide to visit a neighbour.

We can't do this with our feet alone. They won't move by themselves. We have to communicate our desire to take a walk to our brain. Our brain passes the message on to our feet.

The message to walk to the neighbour's house is transmitted by an electrical impulse originating in one or more cells. This impulse passes from the dendrites, through the axon, and on into the terminal shoots or branches that pop out through the end of the axon to the synapse. Once the electrical impulse from our message reaches this synapse, it somehow has to bridge it and communicate with the dendrite receivers of a neighbouring neuron. The impulse does this by stimulating the release of chemicals called *neurotransmitters*. There are many different neurotransmitters. One very important one is *acetylcholine*. Acetylcholine is believed to be responsible for, or plays a major role in, thinking and remembering, and is especially important in the processing of recent or short-term memory.[1]

Once the neurotransmitters are released, they pass through the synaptic space and are attached to the surface of the dendrite receivers at specific locations known as *receptors*. This stimulates the release of a high-energy chemical that switches on the electrical impulse in the next neuron along the path.

The brain then tells our feet to take a walk.

This process of message transmission in the brain is indeed beautiful, rather like a well-crocheted afghan. It is evidence that the brain, like the rest of us, is fearfully and wonderfully made, a complex creation knit together by a loving and imaginative Creator, enabling us to function in amazing ways.

What Goes Wrong?

◄◄ *I tried to explain it to him so he would understand. I told my husband that having Alzheimer's was like having a car with its wires disconnected. I told him they hadn't figured out a way yet to reconnect the wires in his brain. He seemed to accept that.*

◄◄ *I think my son described it best. He said there's a whole lot of switches in the brain and, one by one, they go.*

◄◄ *My husband started acting really strangely in the summer of 1979. By November he was worse. I tried to get him to go to the doctor but he refused.*

He would always shower in the morning. If he was active, he'd shower at midday. He'd also shower at night. But that autumn he let himself go and didn't shower at all. He wouldn't even change his clothes. He seemed deeply depressed.

If I said anything to him about what he was doing, or not doing, he would get angry. I knew there was something wrong, and he knew there was something wrong, but he wouldn't admit it.

One day our son happened to be visiting. He said, 'You

*know, some of the things you're doing aren't you. Don't you
think Mother ought to make an appointment for you to see
a doctor?'*

*I guess my husband needed to hear it from our son,
because he came back into the house later that day and
said, 'You're right. I've got to see a doctor. I've got to find
out what's wrong with me.'*

The year was 1906. The country was Germany.

He was a psychiatrist and neuropathologist. She was a middle-aged housewife who had experienced profound memory loss, language deficits, disorientation, confusion, depression, insomnia, paranoia and hallucinations.

She was his patient. She died in a mental asylum in Frankfurt at the age of fifty-five. After her death, Dr Alois Alzheimer, who was then working at Munich medical school, presented the results of a post-mortem examination.

When Dr Alzheimer looked in his microscope and, using a special silver stain, examined a slice of his patient's brain tissue, he discovered two startling abnormalities, inside and outside the brain cells.

Tissue lying inside the cell bodies or nuclei of neurons exhibited an abnormally high number of fine nerve fibres, or filaments, twisted around each other. Dr Alzheimer called these twisted fibres *neurofibrillary tangles*.

He also saw unusually high numbers of plaques located between brain cells, composed of degenerating terminal dendrites or burned-out nerve endings that contained dead cells and deposits of amyloid protein. These abnormalities were known as *senile* or *neuritic plaques*. They had been identified before in the autopsied brain tissue of much older people.

For many years after 1906, it was believed that this characteristic tangle and plaque configuration occurred primarily in people under the age of sixty; Alzheimer's disease was thought to be a 'pre-senile dementia'. Anyone exhibiting signs of confusion after the age of sixty or sixty-five was simply labelled 'senile', or was said to have a chronic organic brain syndrome, more commonly known as COBS. This senility of old age was universally blamed on faulty blood circulation or so-called hardening of the arteries, and it was thought to be due to an atherosclerotic process of cholesterol build-up in the arteries of the brain.

But in succeeding years, research finally caught up with reality. In the 1960s, as British researchers began comparing the brains of younger, deceased dementia victims with those of older victims, the electron microscope proved what many had suspected all along: the primary cause of dementia-like symptoms in both younger and older victims was, in fact, one and the same. And it wasn't as rare a phenomenon as previously thought.

Investigators believed the fibrous plaques and neurofibrillary tangles disrupted the passage of neurochemical signals between neurons, resulting in memory loss and impaired thought processes.

In general, the greater the amount of plaques, tangles and associated cellular death, the greater the degree of disturbance in intellectual function. These changes in the brain took place over time and were responsible for the progressive nature of the disease. And while there was a decrease in blood flow to the brain in victims of Alzheimer's disease, this decrease was not caused by atherosclerosis but by brain-cell death brought on by the Alzheimer's process.

In the 1970s, researchers discovered another abnormality associated with Alzheimer's disease, one specifically related to neurochemical changes and the neurotransmitter acetylcholine, normally manufactured in the brain by an enzyme known as *choline acetyltransferase*.

In autopsied brain tissue of people who have the characteristic plaques and tangles, choline acetyltransferase and acetylcholine are reduced or present in decreased amounts. Without the stimulus for neurotransmission, signals (messages) are unable to move across the synaptic gap from neuron to neuron. When nerve cells can't communicate with each other, trouble occurs. This neurochemical loss, as well as the appearance of plaques and tangles, occurs primarily in two areas of the brain: the cortex and the hippocampus.

The cortex, or outer surface of the brain's cerebrum, is composed of those cell bodies that enable us to reason, remember and speak. In addition to experiencing the neurochemical loss, the cortex of Alzheimer's victims usually shrinks or atrophies, decreasing the brain's surface area.

The hippocampus is a small cluster of cells located in the temporal lobe. It is extremely important to short-term memory function and is also part of the limbic system. This system, activated by motivated behaviour and arousal, influences both the hormones and the autonomic motor system, which controls involuntary body functions. It has been called 'the seat of our emotions'.

What is actually responsible for the development of plaques and tangles, and the death of acetylcholine-producing cells, is unknown. Researchers around the world are exploring possible causes or combinations of causes that include genetic factors, a slow virus, abnormalities in the immune system, infectious agents, toxic substances in the environment, metabolic deficits and abnormalities in DNA repair. Appendix C includes a more detailed overview of research related to causation.

Alzheimer's disease is more specifically referred to as either a pre-senile dementia or senile dementia of the Alzheimer's type, depending on the age of onset. The former usually occurs before the age of sixty-five; the latter, after the age of sixty-five.

Our brains are indeed awesomely and wonderfully made, but sometimes things do go wrong with this complex computer that controls us – things we struggle to understand.

Seeing the Symptoms

'Hindsight is always better than foresight,' acknowledged one carer. 'I think the reason I didn't see my wife's symptoms earlier was because I was with her all the time. The changes were so subtle, so gradual.'

Probably the most remarkable thing about the very early stages of Alzheimer's disease is its unremarkableness. Signs and symptoms seem to creep up and take us unaware, surprising both us and our loved ones. With the passage of time, the mental and physical deterioration of Alzheimer's becomes more and more pronounced.

While no two people progress at the same rate or according to the same exact pattern, there are some characteristic behaviour and personality changes peculiar to each stage of the illness. Knowing what these changes are can help you promote a better quality of life for both yourself and your loved one. Understanding the signs and symptoms of Alzheimer's is a crucial key to caring.[2]

Two to four years is the average length of the first stage of Alzheimer's. The initial symptoms of Alzheimer's may include any or all of the following changes:

• *Memory loss.* Recent events are forgotten. The ability to concentrate, learn new things and process new information is progressively lost. Bills go unpaid or are paid several times. Bank accounts are overdrawn when the person has trouble adding, subtracting and balancing a cheque book. The names of known and loved persons may also be forgotten.

People with Alzheimer's usually compensate, initially, by writing notes to themselves. But as the disease progresses, they no longer remember the notes. People frequently deny experiencing these symptoms or rationalize them away as they struggle to preserve their self-esteem and identity.

• *Confusion and disorientation.* Confusion is often related to place and time. People with Alzheimer's sometimes get lost on their way somewhere, or they will arrive at a place and not know where they are or how to get home. The day and month are forgotten as well.

• *Speech and language disturbances.* There may be a progressive inability to name objects or to end sentences. The person searches for words and phrases. Wrong words and phrases are substituted for forgotten right ones, a condition known as *confabulation. Circumlocution* may also occur, where more words than necessary are used to express an idea.

• *Impaired judgement.* There's a lack of insight and a growing inability to discriminate, understand and follow directions. Driving is progressively impaired; the person may go through stop signs or end up going the wrong way on one-way streets. The ability to read is retained but not the ability to understand what is read.

• *Difficulty completing familiar tasks.* It becomes increasingly difficult to cook, clean, engage in familiar hobbies or hold down a job. Routine activities of daily living go through a process of 'unlearning'. For example, the ability to tie shoes, button a blouse or shirt, or make a cup of tea or coffee may be impaired.

• *Personality and mood changes.* Depression frequently accompanies the early stage of Alzheimer's. There may be listlessness, apathy, suspiciousness, paranoia, social withdrawal and episodes of crying. Conversely, there may be restlessness, anxiety, agitation, and feelings of 'going crazy'. On the one hand, people deny the severity of their symptoms, while on the other, they recognize that something's wrong.

• *Carelessness and neglect.* Personal hygiene can become a problem, and people may appear careless or unkempt. They may neglect to bathe, brush their teeth, change or wash their clothes. They simply may have forgotten how.

Following a diagnosis, carers usually ask their GP, 'How long do we have? How many months or years?' There is always a need to know.

The time from the onset of Alzheimer's to the person's death varies greatly. It may be a few years or over twenty, depending on any number of other health-related factors. Generally speaking, the younger a person is, the faster the progression and deterioration.

Facing the Second Stage

'There are some lucid moments, but they are few and far between and they seem to be getting farther and farther away from each other,' reported one carer whose wife had been diagnosed with Alzheimer's five years earlier.

As Alzheimer's disease progresses, early stage one symptoms intensify. Memory loss becomes more profound. Behaviour becomes more disturbing, bizarre and unpredictable. This second stage of Alzheimer's may last for between two and ten years.

We need to keep in mind that not all victims of Alzheimer's will experience the same symptoms, but there are some behaviour changes common to dementia.

• *Continued and progressive memory loss.* Past events as well as recent ones may no longer be remembered. The ability to engage in familiar hobbies or carry out even the routine activities of daily living, such as bathing, dressing and toileting, is impaired.

• *Progressive to complete disorientation and confusion.* Our loved ones may lose their ability to recognize people, including family members. They may not recognize their own reflection in a mirror. They may forget the names and uses of familiar objects. They may wander off and get lost, or they may even get lost in their own homes.

• *Speech, communication and language disorders.* People with second-stage Alzheimer's are progressively unable to express themselves and to complete sentences. The repetition of words, questions and phrases is common. Speech may become garbled or very slow.

• *Catastrophic reactions.* These may include pronounced mood swings or personality changes, including outbursts of anger, increased suspiciousness or paranoia, and even episodes of physical violence, usually short-lived.

• *Wandering, restlessness and pacing.* Restless wandering often occurs at night or in the late afternoon, around sundown. Repetitious movements, such as finger or foot tapping, lip smacking and constant chewing motions, may increase.

• *Various behaviour problems.* There may be hallucinations or delusions of being persecuted. People with Alzheimer's frequently hide and hoard things and may tear the house apart looking for 'lost' items. There may be inappropriate sexual and social behaviour with marked social withdrawal.

• *Physical signs.* Motor activity may be affected; many people in the second stage progressively lose their ability to engage in activities requiring hand and finger coordination. Opening a tin with a tin opener, buttoning a shirt, tying a shoelace, hammering a nail – all could be affected. Occasionally there is muscle twitching or jerking. People may tend to lose their balance and fall as coordination becomes impaired. Eating and elimination problems manifest themselves.

Late-stage symptoms include an intensification of stage two symptoms that gradually progress into a need for total care. This stage includes severe cognitive decline. Much supervision and assistance will be needed initially for all activities of daily living. Generally there is progressive incontinence of urine and stool. The ability to walk without assistance may be lost and reflexes can become abnormal due to muscle rigidity. Swallowing may also become impaired, placing the person at risk of dehydration, malnutrition and often pneumonia related to aspiration. Severe or late-stage Alzheimer's disease can last for several years with appropriate supportive care in the home or nursing home. The last chapter of this book discusses the care needs of people in the final stage of Alzheimer's.

The following chapters highlight some of the more common and difficult management problems carers have identified, along with suggestions for dealing with these problems in the varying stages of the disease.

PART TWO

Caring for Your Loved One

We can do no great things –
only small things with great love.

MOTHER TERESA

Chapter Five

When Memory Starts to Fade

'The gifts of God for the people of God. Take them in remembrance that Christ died for you, and feed on him in your hearts by faith, with thanksgiving.'

Father Joe walked slowly down the row of communicants, pausing before each of his parishioners to say the familiar words. 'The body of Christ, the bread of heaven. The body of Christ, the bread of heaven. The body of Christ, the bread of heaven.'

When he came to the last kneeling person, he paused and smiled. Here was Mary again, just as she had been for the past eight months.

Mary. An elderly woman who had never married, and a founder member of the church. A Sunday school teacher for forty years until she was sixty-five, at which time she told everyone she was tired, retired and ready to relax. 'You folks take over,' said Mary. 'I'll sit and enjoy church.'

Mary's habits for the past eight months had become rather unusual. She had developed a weekly pattern of bringing her luggage – two overstuffed suitcases held together with string and adhesive tape – to church. She'd even carry them up to the altar and set them down, one on each side of her. Father Joe once asked Mary where she was going with her suitcases. Mary glared at him and told him it was none of his business.

Today, Mary wasn't exactly dressed for church, not for church on a warm summer morning, at any rate. She had on her bulky grey overcoat with the unravelling hem and what appeared to be several layers of thick wool stockings. A pair of fur-lined boots graced her feet. One toe stuck out through a hole.

It wasn't as though Mary had to wear these clothes, thought Father Joe. The ladies of the church had offered to take her shopping. They'd even purchased some new summer clothes for her and had delivered them n person. But Mary wouldn't let them in the house, telling them she didn't accept charity and to please give the clothes to the poor. 'I'm fine,' Mary insisted. 'Fine.'

And Mary was fine, to a point. The Meals-on-Wheels programme delivered a hot lunch to her – so she was at least eating a balanced midday meal. But Mary never let the volunteers in the house, insisting they leave the food wrapped in a brown paper bag on the porch. By the following morning the previous day's meals had disappeared, and the dirty dishes were back in the paper bag on the porch.

The district nurses were aware of Mary's situation and were also trying to help. They sent a home help to clean her house, but Mary wouldn't let her inside. She insisted, through the keyhole, that she was fine. 'My house is clean,' she told the woman.

'It didn't smell fine and clean through the keyhole!' the home help told her supervisor. 'But what could I do?'

Today, though, Mary's clothes and Mary's house really didn't matter. Mary was here in church, and she was ready to receive communion.

As Father Joe bent down to place the wafer in Mary's mouth, he thought he could detect the faint odour of urine floating up and mingling its ammonia with the aroma of burning incense.

But Mary wasn't aware of this. Her eyes were closed in an attitude of prayer. Her mouth was open to receive the wafer. And her hands gripped the handles of her two packed suitcases.

Of all of us gathered here today, thought Father Joe, Mary is probably the most prepared to enter the heavenly kingdom.

The Faces of Memory Loss

Several weeks before I completed the final draft of the first edition of this book, the father of a member of our support group died. I went to the viewing at the funeral parlour, where my friend and I stood next to her father's coffin, talking about the final, emotionally charged days of his life.

As I was about to leave, my friend turned to me and said, 'Be sure to tell people that Alzheimer's is more than a little memory loss. It's not just forgetting names or how to balance your cheque book.

It's forgetting everything, eventually. Everything you ever did that was important to who you were as a person. Everyone you've ever known. Write about that. People need to know.'

My friend was right. People do need to know. For with knowledge comes understanding and the ability to empathize with carers who have a responsibility that may last anywhere from one to over twenty years. As carers ourselves, we need knowledge and understanding to be able to deal with the many faces of Alzheimer's, especially the many faces of memory loss.

My own mother was an artist. Not a professional artist, but an artist nonetheless. My most vivid childhood memories are of Mum sitting in her living room rocking chair each evening in front of an old easel my father had made, surrounded by little tubes of oil paint or boxes of pastels. Mum was always in the middle of a painting project.

Later in life my mother packed up her paints and pastels and switched to crocheting. With her artist's eye she wove thousands of granny squares into dozens of beautiful afghans. When she first started having symptoms of Alzheimer's, she continued to crochet. In fact, her afghans were one of the first signs that anything was wrong.

I came home for a visit one Christmas and Mum had one of her latest creations spread out on the bed. It basically looked okay, much the same as all her other variegated blue-and-white afghans. This one, however, also contained a few isolated squares of green and white. When I mentioned it, my mother just shrugged. 'Looks okay to me,' I remember her saying. That did not show an artist's appraising eye, and it was not her usual attitude. My mother always liked her afghans to be perfect, and she would tear them apart and start them over if they weren't.

As the months passed, Mum continued to crochet, but the granny squares gradually became circles, then chains and, finally, bunches of tangled wool. Unlike many people with Alzheimer's who become frustrated with the loss of their ability to continue to engage in well-loved hobbies, Mum seemed content to do what she could and was generally oblivious to the fact that her abilities were deteriorating.

◀◀ *My husband forgot how to dress himself. He couldn't figure out how to button his shirt, tie his shoes or buckle his belt. He just couldn't seem to figure out what went where.*

◀◀ *Dad had a colostomy and had always done his own irrigating, but it got to the point where he couldn't remember how to do it. So my mother started to do it for him. Then, eventually, the district nurse came in because Dad wouldn't let my mother touch him.*

◀◀ *The hardest part each morning was trying to brush Mum's teeth. She simply couldn't figure out what to do with the toothbrush. I'd put some toothpaste on the brush and try to show her what I wanted her to do but after a while it was useless. I had to brush them for her if I wanted them brushed at all.*

One of the most difficult and painful behaviour changes carers have to face is the loss of their loved one's memory of self as they fail to recognize themselves.

◀◀ *One morning my mother was sitting in her rocking chair in the bedroom while I cleaned out a cupboard in the hall. All of a sudden I heard her crying and rushed into the bedroom to see what was the matter. She was looking in the mirror repeating the same phrase over and over again: 'I lost myself. I lost myself.'*

No less painful is the realization that our loved one doesn't seem to know us and may have delusions that we are someone else.

◀◀ *I remember one day my mother said to my dad, 'She wants me to sit down. Who is she? Do you know who she is?'*
    If there was anything left of my heart to break, it broke right there. I walked into our back garden and cried my eyes out.

⏮ It got to the point when my father didn't recognize my mother. He thought she was a stranger and would lock her out of the house.

If their dog needed to go out at night, my mother had to go out of the kitchen door and onto the porch to let the dog out of the porch door. Sometimes Dad would get up and lock the kitchen door behind her, and then he wouldn't let her back in.

Twenty-four hours a day she had to wear a skeleton key around her neck.

⏮ My wife finally decided I didn't belong to her. I wasn't her husband. I had no business being in the bedroom with her.

She would rant and rave and carry on about the strange man in her room and kept telling me she didn't have to sleep in the same room with a man.

I told her I wouldn't touch her, that I was just there if she needed help, but she said she didn't need me and was perfectly able to take care of herself.

I used to have to wait until she was asleep to go to bed myself. Do you know how that made me feel?

Some people with Alzheimer's retain some recognition of themselves far into the disease but have no idea who others are or where they are. Many continue to live in memories of the past.

Anna Wilcox resided on the skilled unit of a nursing home where I worked. She was always certain of her identity, if not the time or the place. If you asked her name, she'd declare with authority and in a very loud voice, 'My name is Anna Wilcox!' But if you asked her if she knew where she was, she'd usually say she was in Ohio, teaching a class of fifteen students in a one-room schoolhouse. The year was somewhere around 1939.

In the evenings after I'd given her her medication and turned out her light, she'd tell me about the school. I didn't try to reorient her to reality. At Anna's stage of dementia, reality orientation usually doesn't work. It only frustrates. So instead, I asked her to tell me about the school in Ohio and the children she had taught. And she did.

Often Anna didn't make much sense. She rambled a lot and sometimes mixed up her role as a schoolteacher with her role as a waitress, another job she apparently held for a time. But it really didn't matter at 9:00 p.m. at night. I'd rub her back a little and listen to her stories. Soon she'd be fast asleep with a smile on her face, dreaming, I like to think, about the past.

Simple Memory Joggers

There are many faces of memory loss connected with Alzheimer's disease. As carers we need to accept and acknowledge them, then help our loved ones to deal with them one by one, a day at a time, as the disease progresses.

Here are a few suggestions. Some of these initial ideas can be utilized with the loved one who is still living at home in the early stages of the disease. Others can be helpful as the disease progresses and the ability to read and comprehend written instructions is lost.

• A large wall calendar can help a person keep track of time. Hang a marker nearby so the days can be crossed off as they pass.

• Provide a simple list of the day's activities in the order in which they should occur. For example, 1. Eat breakfast. 2. Take green pill with milk. 3. Feed cat.

Post the list in a conspicuous place.

• Some people with early dementia prefer note cards with memory-jogging information on them about tasks to complete, phone numbers to remember, and so on. These can be kept in a small file box with dividers for different subjects.

• If telling the time is a problem, consider switching to digital clocks. It's easier to read the time than to figure it out. This technique completely cured my mother of asking 'What time is it?' literally dozens of times a day, and it greatly relieved her stress and anxiety. We put digital clocks in the bedroom, living room and kitchen. For some memory-impaired people, however, the reverse is true; an old-fashioned clock face is easier to read.

• Pill boxes labelled for the day of the week and the time of day are available in some chemists. These can be effective in the early stages of Alzheimer's if your loved one, though still able personally to take medication, might mix up pill bottles. If you as a family member fill these you should closely monitor them to make sure your loved one is taking them appropriately.

• Avoid moving things around in the house. Having things in familiar places is an aid to memory, as is keeping to a familiar routine.

• Pictures and/or labels may help a person identify various rooms in the house. For example, if your loved one has trouble finding the bathroom, colour code the door or put a sign on it identifying it as the bathroom. As the disease progresses you may need to switch to a picture of a bath or toilet.

• Some nursing homes have the names or photographs of confused residents outside their rooms. You might also do this in the home. If your loved one can no longer recognize a personal photograph, hang some type of identifying article of clothing such as an old familiar hat or sweater. My mother began to identify her bedroom when we hung a picture of her grandmother and grandfather next to the door. Prior to that, she kept getting lost.

• Labels on various items in the home – hot and cold water taps and the contents of drawers – can also help jog the memory. Again, as the disease progresses, you might switch from large written labels to pictures of actual drawer contents.

• Let *habit* help you. Your loved one may still be able to perform many routine tasks of daily living with a little help from you. Often the problem lies in initiating the activity. Once it is started, habit seems to take over, and routine tasks can continue to be carried out. For example, you may have to put the toothpaste on the brush, hold the brush to your relative's mouth and begin brushing. He or she then may be able to finish the job. Or you may have to cut up food, place some food on a fork and guide hand to mouth a couple of times until the connection is made. Help your loved one maintain independence for as long as possible for both your sakes.

Maintaining People Awareness

• Spend time with your loved one reminiscing. Reminiscence, or 'life review', is a technique frequently used in adult homes and nursing homes for older people without dementia. It may also be a helpful intervention for people in the early stages of dementia.

Talking about people and events from the past, flipping through old photo albums, reading aloud old letters from friends and relatives, looking at old mementoes – all of these activities can help maintain some awareness of self and others. They can also serve to draw you and your loved one closer together. Old familiar songs or hymns that have been an important part of your loved one's life can be used in all stages of the disease. This 'music therapy' can be particularly valuable in the later stages, especially at night.

• Trying to convince people with Alzheimer's that you aren't who they think you are, or that you are who they think you aren't, is probably futile. It may simply provoke a catastrophic or emotional reaction. During non-stressful times, however (and there will be many), remind your loved one of who you are. Say his or her name frequently, too. Our names are important. They're part of our identity. For Alzheimer's sufferers, they can quickly be lost.

• The Alzheimer's sufferer may revert, at various times, to living in the past. As the disease progresses, trying to reorient to reality may no longer work. A better approach may often be to help your loved one focus attention on events from the past and the feelings associated with them.

We all live in the past to a certain extent. We all spend some time daily remembering various events, both good and bad, that were important to us. These events evoke memories and feelings that make us glad or sad. We might assume that the same happens to our loved ones. Instead of getting upset and trying to orient them to the present, we need to help them focus on these events. They may need to talk about them and express their feelings.

One of the most helpful books for professional and family carers is Naomi Feil's *The Validation Breakthrough*, which gives simple techniques for communicating with people with dementia of the Alzheimer's type, especially the very old. It is filled with case studies from Feil's own experience as a gerontological social worker. The focus of this type of therapy is on learning how to enter into the feelings and emotional world of the other person by being an empathetic listener, maintaining a nonjudgemental attitude, and understanding and accepting *their* view of reality rather than imposing our own – all valuable tools for carers.[1]

Thingamajigs and Thingamabobs

Two of my mother's favourite words when I was growing up were *thingamajig* and *thingamabob*. You could always use those words if necessary if you couldn't remember the name of something. They were handy words. We liked them.

As Mum's disease progressed, virtually everything became a 'thingamajig' or a 'thingamabob'. It became increasingly difficult for her to name familiar objects, to complete sentences and, finally, to communicate any thoughts whatsoever.

Language loss as well as memory loss is common in Alzheimer's disease. One frequent behaviour pattern is the substitution of wrong words for right words, especially at the end of a sentence.

◄◄ *One of the first symptoms we noticed early in the progression of my wife's disease was word substitution. This continued for a long time. She'd say something like 'I need to go out and get the bird' when she meant she had to go out and get the mail. Or she needed to 'cook the car' when she meant she needed to cook dinner. I could usually figure out what she meant, but she confused a lot of other people.*

Some people can manage to express a few words of a sentence but not the complete thought. Their communication may sound as if they are reading out of a children's primer in which all the words are nouns and verbs.

⏮ *My husband's conversation became short and clipped. He'd say 'go' when he wanted to go for a ride, 'eat' when he was hungry, and 'love' when he wanted to hug or be hugged.*

Repetitive or perseverative speech is a frequent problem and, for carers, can be one of the most annoying symptoms of the disease. Words, phrases and questions are often repeated over and over again.

⏮ *My wife kept repeating herself until I thought I'd go crazy. Sometimes it was the same word. But the worst thing was the same question – 'What time is it? What time is it? What time is it?' And I always felt I had to answer her.*

Sometimes people with dementia revert to the language of their youth:

⏮ *In the nursing home my father reverted to his childhood language. His mother came from Czechoslovakia and they always spoke the Bohemian language at home. For one period of time, when he was still able to talk, he kept bouncing back and forth between English and Bohemian. It drove the nurses crazy.*

The ability to complete sentences may be lost.

⏮ *My wife would start a sentence. She'd get three or four words out, and the rest was just gibberish. It used to make me feel so bad because I didn't know what she was trying to tell me. She looked so earnest. I would say, 'Is that right?' And that seemed to please her even though it didn't satisfy me.*

⏮ *Once in a while a word comes out I can understand, like 'Christmas', or a phrase like 'It's cold in here.' But most of the time my husband just babbles. Sometimes we sit and babble together. I love to hear his voice. I dread the day when his babbling stops. Can you understand that?*

Eventually language may fail altogether.

◄◄ *Now my father can't even form words to talk to me. It's like his tongue is three times its normal size. He tries to say something once in a while but no intelligible word will come out.*

If I say, 'Dad, are you okay?' he may shake his head yes or no. Then again, he may not.

Breaking Through the Walls

Language losses are not easy to deal with, but the following tips may help facilitate both the giving and receiving of information as you learn new ways to communicate.

• Face your loved one when speaking and maintain eye contact. Speak slowly and distinctly and lower the pitch of your voice. This is especially important if there is any hearing impairment. A low voice is more important than a loud voice.

• Ask questions or give directions one at a time. Don't expect immediate responses. Give the person you care for time to process the information before answering or actively responding. If he or she is trying to respond verbally but is becoming frustrated, help out. You may need to finish a sentence or supply a word. Help to decrease anxiety.

• Tune in to your loved one's body language. Listen to what is being said via facial expressions, body movements, posture and so forth. If an Alzheimer's sufferer is trying to communicate something but can't verbally express it, try asking simple questions that can be answered with yes, no or a head movement. If you suspect he or she is in pain, you may have to point to or touch the area you think might be hurting. Ask for a response with a nod of the head, to see if you are correct.

• There are no sure cures for repetitious verbalizations and behaviours, though looking for possible contributing causes is always a first step. For example, 'oh, oh, oh' repeated over and over may be because of pain or the need to go to the toilet.

Sometimes you can determine no underlying reason for the behaviour, even though your loved one seems anxious and troubled. If you say 'It's okay' or 'It's all right' and show affection, you may help the sufferer feel less anxious and more secure.

Music may also be helpful for curbing repetition. Sarah White, a nursing-home resident diagnosed with Alzheimer's, constantly tapped her foot on the floor and her fingers on the arm of her wheelchair. She also repeated, 'I'm lost, I'm lost, I'm lost.' One day we discovered that Sarah had been a minister's wife and a minister's daughter. Church attendance had been a regular part of her life, but no one knew it at the home. When we discovered this, we began taking her to weekly church services. As soon as she heard the music playing and the congregation singing, Sarah stopped her repetitious tapping, except to keep time to the music. She also stopped saying, 'I'm lost.'

We finally got a radio for Sarah's room and kept it tuned to a religious or a classical music station. The music seemed to soothe her, and the repetitious, perseverative behaviour and verbalizations diminished.

If all your attempts to intervene and break the cycle of repetition fail, you may have to simply remove yourself from the scene for a while to keep from blowing your cool. Pray for patience to weather it until next time.

The many faces of memory loss are indeed painful to see, but the losses can be lessened as we look for ways to preserve and enhance the memory that still exists.

Chapter Six

Emotional Fireworks

◄◄ *We never fought when I was growing up. My mother was very sweet, gentle and easygoing. But we fought when she got Alzheimer's.*

One dictionary definition of *catastrophe* is 'a sudden, violent change, such as an earthquake'. This well describes the various catastrophic reactions that frequently accompany Alzheimer's, ranging from the slight tremor of anxiety to a sometimes violent verbal or physical outburst.

Catastrophic reactions are hard to understand. A closer look, however, can often indicate some underlying reasons for our loved one's bizarre behaviour. We need to be aware of the various pressure points that might suddenly trigger an emotional eruption.

Triggers for Catastrophic Reactions

Catastrophic reactions can occur when an Alzheimer's sufferer is frustrated by diminishing abilities.

◄◄ *My dad had been an excellent mechanic. But it got to the point where he ruined everything he touched. It was the most pitiful thing to see.*

I'll never forget one experience. Dad's Jeep was sitting in the garage and he was tinkering with it, trying to get it to run. He finally came running into the house, absolutely beside himself.

'I can't do it,' he was crying. 'I can't do it. Would you fix my Jeep? Would you fix my Jeep?' That broke my heart.

Reactions can sometimes be triggered by irrational fears. They may be accompanied by paranoia.

◀◀ *The district nurse would try to give my husband a bath or even just wash him, and he'd fight. You couldn't struggle with him because you'd lose. He had the strength of a bull. He wouldn't let anyone near him. He'd say that the water was cold, that he was afraid of it.*

◀◀ *My mother was absolutely terrified one evening, and she kept pointing to the double door on our deck. I was sure someone was out there, but then I realized she was seeing her own reflection in the glass. I remembered to keep the curtains closed after that episode.*

◀◀ *Once, when my mother was still driving, she looked in the rearview mirror and really got hysterical. She was sure the person in the car behind us was following us.*
The person in the car was my brother!

Catastrophic reactions can sometimes be triggered by specific actions on the part of another person, especially if the other person is perceived as a threat in any way.

◀◀ *If my father felt threatened he would pinch or hit, especially if you tried to get him to do something he didn't want to do.*

◀◀ *One night I had to take my mother to the hospital for a medical emergency, and a friend of mine stayed with my father.*
My father kept wanting to go to the hospital too, and he tried to get in the car. He hit my friend over the head with a torch three times when she tried to stop him.

Reactions can occur when we try to get our loved one to choose from various options or respond to several questions at once.

◀◀ *I remember taking my father to restaurants. I was trying to make him feel better about himself, so I would always ask him to choose what he wanted to eat; I wanted to give him a choice. But instead of feeling better he became frustrated and upset because there were too many things to choose from. He couldn't process all that information, and once he even started to cry. When I finally understood what was happening, we still went out, but I simply ordered for us both.*

Catastrophic reactions usually seem like marked personality changes. They are sometimes accompanied by outpourings of profanity and verbal abuse, directed at us. Occasionally they turn into physical violence.

⏮ *My husband got nasty, really nasty, and he was never nasty in his life. He even punched me once with his fists.*

⏮ *One minute my wife seems to know who we are, and five minutes later she'll be yelling and calling us names. It's just as if somebody turns a switch and another person appears. She gets violent and very abusive, just the opposite of what she used to be.*

She was one of the most lovable people. There wasn't enough she could do for other people. And she never swore. But since she's developed Alzheimer's, I've learned language from her I didn't know existed.

It's a natural tendency to respond to our loved one's catastrophic reactions with emotional outbursts of our own. Catastrophic reactions are stressful and emotionally charged experiences, and if we're feeling unduly stressed to begin with, we will react rather than respond. But if we do that, we're in for trouble. As soon as the episode is over, we'll feel like a failure because of the way we handled the situation.

The key phrase to remember when confronted with a catastrophic reaction on the part of a loved one is *keep calm*. That may seem difficult, if not impossible, to do given the circumstances, but it is the best advice we can give ourselves. It will help to divert disaster and convert catastrophes into experiences we and our loved ones will be able to live through.

What to Do and What to Avoid

The following dos and don'ts offer some practical suggestions:

• Do avoid situations or events that might trigger catastrophic reactions. If you can't avoid them, anticipate them. For example, if you take your loved one food shopping, avoid Saturday mornings and Friday nights. Go at times when the supermarket is less likely to be a hive of people. If you go out to eat, avoid the prime-time hours when restaurants are crowded.

• Do make life as predictable as possible. Most of us get tired of the same old grind, but people with dementia find a daily routine secure and comfortable. Marked schedule changes may precipitate catastrophic reactions. Plan your loved one's life as much as possible. This may become less of a problem as the disease progresses.

• Do limit choices. Remember that your loved one's ability to discriminate is markedly affected by Alzheimer's. If you are helping your mother or wife to dress, for example, asking her to choose from the blue, brown, yellow or white dress may overwhelm her. Instead, you could show her two dresses and ask her to choose one. Or you may simply have to choose one for her.

Use simple sentences. Offer one thought at a time. Let one task be completed before talking about another one.

• Do simplify the activities of daily living. In the area of clothing, consider substituting pullover dresses, shirts and sweaters for those that button; slip-on shoes for those with laces; and Velcro fasteners for zippers, buttons and poppers. Such replacements will help your loved one maintain independence for as long as possible while minimizing catastrophic reactions.

• Don't talk about your loved one's behaviour problems to others in the presence of your loved one. Just because someone may no longer be able to communicate verbally does not mean he or she no longer understands what's going on or what's being said. Think about how you'd feel in a similar situation and be sensitive. Always assume more understanding and comprehension than you can actually see.

• Don't take personally the things your loved one says. You or other family members may be accused of stealing money, selling the family home or withdrawing your love. Attempting to deny the accusations may only make things worse.

If you are accused of stealing money, for example, you might offer to help your loved one search for it. One carer I interviewed has a locked box for which she keeps the key. Inside the box are her mother's cheque book, recent bank receipts and a little cash. If her mother accuses her of theft, they search for the box together. When they 'find' it, her mother leafs through the bank statements and the cheque book and usually concludes that all is intact. The catastrophic reaction blows over.

• Don't argue or try to reason. Remember that the disease affects the memory and the mind's ability to think logically. Sufferers may not understand why it isn't safe for them to drive the family car. To believe that they will understand if someone just explains it enough times is an error of judgement. Arguments can also make your loved one more suspicious and defensive – attitude changes you don't need.

Instead of arguing and reasoning, acknowledge and validate. The disorientation and confusion that are part of Alzheimer's result in more than just bizarre behaviours. Dementia also stirs up deep feelings – for us *and* our loved ones. These feelings seem to have little to do with intellectual impairment. Beneath a belligerent exterior, our loved ones may be nursing a lot of fear, disappointment and hurt – just as we would if we were frustrated in our attempts to do something we'd always loved to do, something that was an important part of our identity. Helping our loved ones to verbalize those feelings, or even to cry, may be the best thing we can do.

• Do avoid shouting or raising your voice. Don't correct or confront the bizarre behaviour. A loud, accusatory voice implies that we somehow expect change in the behaviour. We need to remember that the behaviour is not deliberate. People with Alzheimer's don't want to act the way they do.

Avoid the 'why' questions: 'Why are you doing this?' or 'Why did you do it?' 'Why' questions can put others on the defensive. They feel they have to justify their behaviour, which in this case they are not responsible for. The normal reaction to a perceived threat is fight or flight. Both are catastrophic reactions. What our loved ones need most is our love and acceptance of who they are, just as they are.

Speak softly, treating the person you care for with the same dignity and respect you would want to be shown if you were in the same shoes. A proverb says, 'A gentle answer quiets anger, but a harsh one stirs it up.' Soothing answers and soft tones can temper many a catastrophic reaction.

• Do move beyond the event and forget it as quickly as possible. Defuse situations by using a technique called distraction. Distraction might include changing the subject, going for a walk to 'search' for the missing item, or offering a favourite food to eat.

Be thankful for your loved one's short-term memory and consider it a blessing in the case of catastrophic reactions.

• Don't physically restrain your loved one. He or she may feel fenced in and become even more combative. Instead, capitalize on the excess energy at this time. If your loved one is turning over the living room furniture, it might be an ideal time to clean the rug! Try to redirect the energy and get him or her to help you.

• Do consider the possibility that medication, such as a mild tranquillizer, may help your loved one. Catastrophic reactions are often like dormant volcanoes – they suddenly erupt without much warning and are over as quickly as they started. But in some cases the catastrophe may seem continuous. If this is the case for you, talk with your doctor about possible medication.

• Do remove yourself from emotionally charged situations. If you feel you are going to explode, you probably will. It's no sin to walk away from your loved one if you think the situation is going to get the better of you, or if you anticipate physical violence. If you can do so without endangering anyone's safety, leave the scene for a time and return when everyone has calmed down.

• Avoid emotionally distancing yourself. Reach out with a warm embrace, a kiss, a touch of your hand. Affection can often defuse a difficult situation. Touch can communicate that you care. It can offer reassurance and affirmation as well as affection.

'Perfect love drives out all fear,' says a verse in the New Testament. Our love for the people we care for may not be perfect. In fact, we may feel very unloving at times. But it will ultimately be our love that will drive out the fears we have – and the fears our loved ones have – in dealing with the various catastrophic reactions of Alzheimer's.

Relying on Rituals

Engaging the person with Alzheimer's in familiar rituals may also be a very helpful intervention. As a nurse working on special care dementia units and as a spiritual care coordinator in one nursing home, I discovered something that should always be assessed when a person was admitted to a home – familiar rituals and practices that had been a daily part of life. Practices associated with a person's faith can be particularly meaningful.

Helen spent most of her day wandering the halls on the special care unit where I worked. She would seldom sit down and when she did it was often on the floor where she leaned against a wall, talking to herself. Late afternoon was the time of day when her agitation and restlessness increased. Helen frequently struck out physically at other nursing home residents if they invaded her personal space, and also at nursing home staff if they tried to intervene. Her agitation was particularly acute following visits from her daughter; Helen always insisted she be allowed to go home. Her daughter often left the nursing home in tears or engaged in an argument with her mother in the hall, which frequently resulted in a catastrophic reaction.

One afternoon Helen saw the lift door open and made a dash for it; she was restrained by two nursing assistants and began to kick and struggle. She was finally settled in a chair by the nurses' station and physically she was quieter, but it was clear her emotional distress was unrelieved. Helen held her head in her hands, rocked back and forth in the chair and kept repeating, 'Oh, no. Oh, dear. Oh, no.'

On the special care unit at the time was a social worker. I was the nurse in charge that evening. As the social worker and I brainstormed possible solutions to help moderate or alleviate Helen's agitated behaviour, the social worker reminded me that Helen was Catholic and said she thought she remembered seeing a rosary in her room. I retrieved the rosary and brought it to Helen. Her response was to grab it out of my hand and then to more carefully hold it, stroke it and begin to recite the words. Within a period of fifteen minutes, Helen was calm and I was able to carry on a very lucid conversation with her. When I asked her if she would like me to pray for her, Helen readily agreed. She clutched the rosary in one hand and held my hand with the other. After the prayer she was visibly calmer. Helen's use of the rosary and my use of prayer became a regular part of nursing care for Helen. Relying on rituals that are important to our loved ones can also be a very effective intervention for carers at home.[1]

Chapter Seven

Always on the Move

I once worked in a nursing home that had a locked unit, in the days before safety devices such as alarm bracelets could be worn by residents to alert staff that someone was close to an exit. All the residents there had some form of dementia, and all were free to roam and wander around, including Sam Smith.

Sam was a man in his eighties. In his younger years he had worked as a guard on the local railway; when Sam stood by the exit door of the ward, he still looked the part. He wore his old battered conductor's cap and carried a paper bag filled with biscuits. 'My lunch,' he'd say, if anyone asked. If anyone questioned why he was waiting by the door at the same time every day, Sam would smile and say, 'Waiting for the train.'

When the evening nurses pressed the buzzer on the outside of the door to signal to the day staff that they had arrived, Sam would get excited. He thought it was the train whistle.

Sam would continue to pace back and forth by the door for an hour after the shift change. Then he'd go back to his room and wait for tomorrow's train.

Sundowning

When the sun goes down, people with Alzheimer's frequently want to get up and go. Confusion heightens at this time of day and into the night. Restless wandering and agitation increase. This phenomenon is called *sundowning* or *sundown syndrome*.

Sundowning is a common occurrence in nursing homes for people with Alzheimer's. It also occurs at home, and it is often accompanied by catastrophic reactions.

⏮ *My wife's restlessness and agitation seem to be worse in the winter months, when it gets dark early in the afternoon.*

> *Sometimes she gets angry along with getting restless
> and agitated. Her anger might last half an hour or four
> or five hours. That big crack in the window over there
> happened late one afternoon when my wife got angry and
> threw her shoe.*

Reasons for sundowning are unclear, though late-afternoon fatigue may be a contributing factor. It's also wise to consider obvious and correctable physical catalysts for odd behaviour: hunger, thirst or the need to go to the bathroom.

If rest, food, drink, or bladder or bowel elimination fail to calm your loved one's agitation, here are some things you can do to cope with it.

Simplify and modify the environment

In nursing homes, sundowning frequently occurs during shift changes, when nurses and assistants are coming and going and causing confusion. Some times of day are more confusing than others in the home as well. For example, a younger person with Alzheimer's who has school-age children may find after-school time particularly stressful. The kids come home with their friends, the TV blares, the house is in an uproar.

You may not be able to change the environment, but you can move your loved one to a room away from busy people traffic. Total isolation isn't always necessary, but quieter surroundings may help decrease stress.

The day-care home where I took my mother every morning for a year so I could work had a very large fenced-in garden where residents could freely and safely walk. Every person reacts differently to being in a more confined area: for many it appears to provide a secure environment where they can safely roam; you might find for others it increases agitation. Experimentation is generally needed.

Low lighting and increased shadows may also be contributing factors that can increase confusion. Night-lights or low-glow lights in certain areas of the home may help reduce agitation.

Find simple things for your loved one to do

One helpful idea comes from a carer in a residential home. She calls it a 'rummage box':

⏮ *I made up what I call Mary's rummage box. Every afternoon Mary would enter other people's rooms in our home and go through their dresser drawers. Needless to say, she wasn't very popular with some of the more alert people.*

I got Mary a big box and filled it with soft things like washcloths, towels, balls of wool and soft toys. Then I sat Mary down at the kitchen table while I got dinner ready. For an hour or so she seemed content just taking the things out of the box one by one and putting them back in. She'd also fold and unfold the towels and facecloths.

Spend time with your loved one

Let him or her be near you. Lack of security may contribute to sundowning. Your loved one may need the reassurance that you, unlike the setting sun, won't leave.

Find easy things to do together that are meaningful and productive: washing and drying dishes, sweeping the floor, emptying the bins, polishing shoes. Activities that a person has engaged in previously are often ingrained as habits. You may need to rewash, resweep, or refold the sheets, but the fact that you're able to continue sharing in these daily activities is worth the extra time.

A person with Alzheimer's may not be able to clean the whole house or cook an entire meal, but the loss of these abilities is usually gradual. You can capitalize on the abilities that are still intact and help preserve them for as long as possible. When you do that, you also help preserve your loved one's self-esteem.

If your relative's behaviour is manageable, perhaps late afternoon is the best time to shop for food, do errands or simply get away from it all. Go for a drive and enjoy the scenery together.

Reliving pleasures from the past may also be a means of calming down a person with Alzheimer's and providing an enjoyable experience. Consider watching an old movie on television, looking through photo albums, and talking about old times and old friends. Sing some favourite songs or hymns. Play the piano. Encourage your loved one to play if they have in the past; people with advanced dementia who have played instruments often still can with very little difficulty, especially if they play by ear. Never underestimate learned abilities. Put on a record and dance. Do what you used to do. Focus on the familiar.

Late afternoon may also be a good time to take a walk with your loved one. It's good exercise for you both, and you might find that an exercise break will decrease nightly wandering and enhance your loved one's ability to sleep. Research also appears to indicate that light morning exercise, including walking, may help to decrease agitation, wandering and aggressive behaviours. An added benefit of twenty to thirty minutes of daytime walking is sunshine. Though there are concerns about too much long-term exposure to sun contributing to the development of skin cancer, sunlight is a significant source of vitamin D which, research indicates, helps to maintain a healthy immune system with normal exposure. Vitamin D also helps to maintain adequate levels of calcium and phosphorus and aids in maintaining strong bones.[1]

Sundowning can indeed cause frustration and anxiety for everyone in the family touched by Alzheimer's disease. But it can also be an incentive for new dimensions of creativity and companionship.

Prone to Wander

You'd think a lot of restless wandering throughout the day would exhaust your loved one as much as it does you, but this is not always the case. Many people with Alzheimer's continue to wander well into the night and on into the early hours of the morning.

⏮ *I was always on the alert. My husband would get up around 2:00 a.m. and turn on the light in our room. He'd pack a suitcase, or sometimes just a box of trinkets, and head downstairs. Sometimes he'd just roll his bedding up and take it downstairs and pile it on the floor. Usually he got dressed.*

So then I'd get out of my bed and put my housecoat on and go downstairs with him, and we'd just sit in the living room chairs in the dark until 4:00 or 5:00 a.m. and then we'd both go back to bed for a while.

He never tried to go out at night, but he was up for most of it.

⏮ *My wife started living in the past, living on the farm where she grew up. She was always getting out of bed in the middle of the night. Then she'd wander all through the house, looking for the animals.*

⏮ *My husband wandered all over the house at night. I stayed awake to make sure he was all right. The doctor wanted me to tie my husband in bed so I could get some rest, but I just couldn't. And the medications he gave him only seemed to make him worse, especially during the day.*

So he wandered and I didn't get much sleep. I finally hired people to stay at night, but that first year was terrible.

If wandering around the house at night is part of your relative's lifestyle, the following suggestions may be helpful. As always with behaviour management issues, think about physical causes first.

• Hunger or thirst can contribute to restless wandering. Your loved one may be looking for food or something to drink. Offer a small glass of warm milk or herbal tea just before retiring. Avoid anything with caffeine, including hot chocolate. Consider the addition of complex carbohydrate foods, such as a sandwich or biscuits and cheese.

• On the other hand, what you perceive as restlessness may be the sign of a full bladder. Be sure there is a visit to the toilet before retiring, and watch out for excessive fluid intake for several hours prior to going to bed. You might also try placing a commode in a strategic spot, either at the foot of the bed or in front of the bedroom door, if finding the bathroom in the middle of the night presents a problem. Night-lights can also help ensure safer passage.

• If your relative suffers from some other malady in addition to Alzheimer's that may cause pain, consider appropriate pain medication at night. Pain can contribute to agitation. Research in nursing homes indicates that people with dementia tend to be under-medicated for pain, which is not always assessed.

• Nightly wandering may also be a symptom of daily inertia. What may be needed during daylight hours to enhance night-time sleep is some sort of *sustained activity,* such as a planned walk or two around the block. One nursing home I worked in had a supervised hour of walking in the early evening for people with dementia.[2] Carers who have built structured walking times into their loved one's routine have commented on improved sleep and less overall restlessness.

• Think about the effect environmental cues might have on confused people. If your loved one gets up at night and spies his coat and hat on the chair and his clothes all neatly laid out for the next morning, he may assume it is already the next morning, get up and get dressed. You might also want to disguise obvious exits with not-so-obvious curtains.

• A warm bath or shower prior to retiring may help your loved one relax. Avoid bubble baths. They can contribute to urinary tract infections, a complication you don't need. Follow the bath with a soothing back rub.

• Keep a bedside radio tuned softly to a classical music station or the type of music your loved one has always enjoyed. Some carers leave the TV turned on low. Experiment if necessary. A chat show may be the perfect soporific.

• Many people have been used to reading a book before retiring. Reading to your loved one from a familiar source can help induce sleep. In one nursing home I worked in one of the medication sheets for an older person with Alzheimer's noted: 'Please read the twenty-third psalm to Mrs Jones after giving her her evening medication.' In another home saying the Lord's Prayer with a resident became part of the nightly routine. Many people with dementia may still be able to read very well themselves, even though comprehension may be compromised. Your loved one may also enjoy reading to you.

• Cuddly things like stuffed toys can be comforting and seem to lend a sense of security to someone with Alzheimer's, especially women, though infection control requirements for nursing homes and hospitals may need to be taken into account and stuffed objects may be discouraged.

• Sleep medication may be the answer for some, but it should generally be used as a last resort. You will need a prescription for most medications. You might ask your doctor for a dosage range and be sure the medication is in a low-enough dose to allow you to experiment. Never use more when less will do. If tranquillizers are taken during the day, you might be able to divide them up so the stronger dose can be given at night, though discussing medication changes with your GP or district nurse is important. Some medications can be cut in half but others should not be. Medications do come in various strengths, however.

Remember that all medications, including sleep medications, have side effects. A medication one person tolerates well can send another person into a tailspin. This is true for over-the-counter sleep medications as well as prescription drugs. Some may even stimulate rather than depress the central nervous system. The pharmacist or chemist who supplied the medication can answer carer questions about drug effects and possible side effects.

• Carers may feel the use of some type of restraint – for example, a vest or waist restraint – might be helpful to discourage wandering. The general rule in hospitals and nursing homes in the US is that restraints can be used only with a doctor's order if the person is in danger of harming themselves – for example, by pulling out a feeding tube. In the UK restraints are not allowed except in extreme situations and then only for a limited period of time based on decisions made by a team of health-care professionals. Injuries related to restraints have resulted in new rulings for nursing homes; most nursing homes no longer use them and rely on careful monitoring instead. Increased agitation, increased infections such as urinary tract infections, and physical de-conditioning have been consequences of restraints on nursing home residents and they do not appear to prevent falls according to the research literature. People with dementia often try to remove them and may injure themselves in the process. Should agitation become an issue, family members who have placed a loved one with advanced dementia in a nursing home should consult with the nursing home staff about specific wishes on the part of their loved one regarding life-prolonging measures and specific care options that would affect interventions like feeding tubes or intravenous solutions. There are a number of options for carers in the home that are also used in nursing homes: sling-seated wheeled devices, bed or chair alarms that are activated when the person starts to rise, and soft chairs with lower seats.

• While it may not be the norm in the UK, some family carers may consider hiring a non-family carer for the night shift to allow them to get some sleep. If you can do this, use the skills of the substitute carers. Remember, you are paying them. They shouldn't be sleeping on the job! This is a very common practice in the US as agency help is often not available for night caring.

Set up a plan with them that will include their responsibilities – for example, a morning routine of bathing, toileting, dressing, shaving, nail care and so on. Let them do the tasks you find difficult to do or that rob you of your needed energy. If your loved one is awake for large blocks of time in the night, some of these activities could be completed then, while you sleep.

• Be aware that some people with Alzheimer's may get up, get dressed, wander around the house for an hour or so, then head for the nearest chair or sofa and promptly fall asleep. Don't worry too much about where they sleep or what they're wearing. The important thing is that they do sleep.

• If, in spite of all your efforts, your loved one is still prone to wander nocturnally, you'll need to provide for safety. Barriers can be created across doors with curtains, for example. Alarms can also be placed on doors to alert carers. Doors may also need to be locked, with keys hidden but readily available to unlock the door in case of emergency. Neighbours should also be made aware of your situation and told about potential wandering behaviour; they may be of valuable assistance to you if your loved one does wander off. (See Chapter Nine for more information about safety issues.)

Leaving Home

Bill Stewart looked out of the kitchen door. The moon hung full, illuminating the path to the road. Helen, Bill's wife, was asleep. She'd locked the kitchen door, just as she always did, but tonight she'd forgotten to remove the key. Bill saw it, turned it and then stepped out into the moonlight.

The town was seven miles north of their farm. Bill turned right at the gate and headed down the lonely country road.

The next morning a frantic Helen and two policemen found Bill curled up on a bench in the centre of town. Sleeping.

Helen and Bill are certainly not alone in their nocturnal experience. People with Alzheimer's frequently wander aimlessly through their homes. Often they wander away from them. Night or day. Of all the bizarre behaviour patterns of persons with Alzheimer's, wandering away from home and getting lost is one of the most disturbing to carers.

◀◀ My husband ran away from home several times. I remember one time when he said he was going to pick blackberries. He took his basket and ran off in the rain. My daughter and I went after him, but we lost him in the woods and had to go back home and call the police.

After we called, we started searching again. We finally found him ourselves, up on the hill. He was soaking wet. And his basket was empty.

◀◀ You see those geraniums there in the window? Well, once when I got home from work my wife had wandered off. I found a couple of cuttings of geraniums along the street and then I found more. I just kept picking up geranium cuttings until I found her. When we got home I put all the cuttings in water. The ones in the window are their descendants.

◀◀ There were two places I usually thought to look for my wife. One was the church. The other was the supermarket. One day she wasn't at either of those places. I looked everywhere and finally I came home.

After I'd been home for a while I got a phone call from my neighbour. He said he'd seen my wife wandering around a car park, and he'd persuaded her to let him bring her home.

When she was well she would never walk away like that. I don't know where she thought she was going. That car park is three miles away.

◀◀ One day Dad ran off into the woods. I spent an hour and a half looking for him. I was about to call the police when he came out of the woods by our house, and they called me.

You know, the feelings of guilt and embarrassment we suffered in the beginning were totally unnecessary. But we didn't know what was happening.

Finally I said to my mother, 'This man is sick. It's

nothing to be ashamed of. Let's tell everybody.' So we
started with the neighbours. I told them all, 'If you see my
father wandering, let me know immediately.'
   It was a good thing we did that.

Wandering off is not confined to wandering away from home.
Sometimes people with Alzheimer's wander away when they're on
holiday.

   ⏮ *Three years ago my family was at a museum up north. In*
   this museum you had to go in and out of different rooms to see
   the different exhibits.
   We'd gone about two-thirds of the way round when we
   suddenly realized my wife wasn't with us. We thought she
   must have come out of one of the rooms and turned in the
   opposite direction from the rest of us.
   We searched. We went all around the building and into
   other buildings. We looked everywhere. Finally we went out
   into the car park, and there she was. She'd gotten into the
   exit queue and wandered out of the gate.
   When we came up to her she said to us, 'Well, I found
   the car, but I couldn't find the keys. If I had found them I'd
   have gone home.'
   And I think she would have. Or tried to.
   That was our first experience of wandering off. There
   have been many more since.

If your loved one wanders away, you are faced with an emergency
situation that could easily turn to tragedy. The phrase to remember
is *don't panic*. The following strategies can help you cope.

• Don't spend time blaming yourself for your loved one's
disappearance. Guilt won't help find anyone. If needed, call for
assistance. Contact neighbours, friends, relatives and the police to
aid in the search. It's also good to let other people in the area know
your loved one is lost. They may not be officially part of the search
party, but they can be on the alert. Think about the obvious places

your loved one might go – especially places familiar in the past – and share your information with the searchers.

• Search parties need a description of the person they're looking for. Have some recent colour photographs at home. Also keep pictures of your loved one in the glove compartment of your car.

• Notify local accident and emergency departments and nursing homes of your loved one's disappearance. If some Good Samaritan finds your loved one wandering down the road, they might take him or her to one of these places. If you are also out looking, be sure someone stays at your home in case your loved one returns.

• Your loved one should have an identification card or a bracelet or necklace that says 'memory impaired', 'memory loss' or 'Alzheimer's disease'. It can also include name, address and your phone number. If the person has a medical condition in addition to Alzheimer's, such as angina or diabetes, that information should be included along with allergies to any medications. Identification (ID) jewellery can be purchased through some jewellers and inexpensively engraved for you. There's a wide range of prices. Wallet-size ID cards may not be a good substitute for an ID bracelet or necklace for some people with Alzheimer's because they can be easily lost or thrown away. The Alzheimer's Society also recommends a Medic-alert bracelet or a similar form of identification if a person with Alzheimer's is travelling or going on holiday with loved ones and wandering off is a possibility.

• Finding your loved one is only half the battle. Now you have to get him or her home. The chances are your loved one will be relieved to see you. They may be upset and know they are lost. On the other hand, you may not be seen as a rescuer but as someone to fend off or hide from.

Whatever the case, stay calm. Avoid running up, pulling on a sleeve or trying to reason. Remind other rescuers that these techniques probably won't work. Instead, you might ask your loved one where he's going and offer to walk with him or take him with you. Most wanderers are looking for home. Home with you is where they really want to be.

If the person you care for is always on the move, don't despair. With foresight, planning and some practical strategies, we can maintain a relatively safe and secure environment for the perpetual or nocturnal wanderer. Technological advances today also include radio transmitters worn by people with dementia that allow them to be located if they wander off. One example of a resource for carers in the UK is WanderGuardian, which uses Global Positioning Satellite (GPS) technology to locate people who may be lost. There is also a UK Wandering Network (UKWN) website, which contains very helpful information for family carers and professionals about issues related to wandering and helpful prevention strategies and resources for carers. (See Appendix D for information.)

Looking for lost loved ones is a challenge most of us have to face at some point. It's a challenge we will meet when that point comes.

Chapter Eight

Baffling Behaviours

My mother often used to take me visiting with her when I was a child. Occasionally we'd go to the homes of relatives who had ornaments and glassware lying around on tables and shelves, just waiting to be knocked off. But my mother had trained me well. I always walked around with my hands either behind my back or in my pockets. So did she!

When Mum developed Alzheimer's, she acted just the opposite, reaching out and touching everything in sight. Sometimes she took the things she touched.

Hoarding

When I used to go food shopping, Mum usually went with me. I would push her ahead of me in her portable wheelchair and pull the shopping trolley behind us. When our shopping was completed, I carefully checked her pockets and the sleeves of her cardigan before checking out. Mum had a tendency, often when I was busy looking in a particular section, to reach out and touch the assortment of packaged cakes and biscuits in the middle of the aisle. If a package was small, colourful and looked good to eat, my mother might pocket it for future consumption.

In a nursing home where I occasionally worked, one resident had the habit of wandering into other people's rooms and rummaging through their drawers, collecting things to 'take home'. I sometimes found her exiting a room carrying a shoe, dentures, a box of paper hankies or underwear.

Asking her to give up these items was like asking a toddler to relinquish a favourite toy. 'No' was always the answer, accompanied by a set jaw and an even firmer grip on the pilfered items. I was usually able to retrieve them, though, if I offered to swap. The swap might take the form of a biscuit, a glass of milk or a magazine. Sometimes it took several exchanges to accomplish the task, but it worked and we both ended up happy. (I found this also worked well with another resident who had a habit of pinching the nursing home fire extinguisher!)

People with Alzheimer's are a little like pirates. In the words of Janet Sawyer of the Blumenthal Jewish Home, Clemmons, North Carolina, they love to 'rummage, pillage and hoard'. Then they may pocket the loot (food, shoes, neckties, jewellery and so forth) and stash it away in a hiding place that they alone seem to know about.

⏮ *It got to the point where everybody was 'stealing' Dad's stuff. He thought people were coming into the house and hiding things from him, but he was really the one who was doing the hiding.*

My father was for ever losing his tool-box. It was his prized possession, so he would hide it – and then forget where he'd hidden it. One of his favourite hiding places was under the china cupboard in the living room. But sometimes the tool-box wound up under the bed or down in the cellar.

He'd say to my mother, 'Where are my tools? What did you do with them?' And, to keep the peace, my mother would have to go with him and search for them.

⏮ *There was this terrible odour coming from my mother's room. The auxiliaries finally worked it out. Mum had tucked away a chicken leg in the drawer of her bedside table.*

How do we solve the problem of taking and losing things? Asking 'Where did you hide it this time?' never works and is demeaning. There are gentle, loving and practical ways to discover where your wife has stashed the family jewels or where your father has hidden the house keys.

• Have a place only you know about to put car keys, cash and other irreplaceable items. Make small and easily lost articles more visible by attaching them to larger and more colourful things, like key rings. Be sure you have duplicates of whatever can be duplicated.

• Put bills and other important papers out of reach and out of sight. Many Alzheimer's sufferers don't just hide things, they also rip them up.

• Check the contents of wastebins before throwing out the rubbish.

• Lock the toilet door if your loved one has a tendency to flush away valuables.

• You may need to lock inner doors, cupboards and drawers. This not only protects other people's valuables but also eliminates hiding places.

• If you're truly stumped, think of some of the not-so-obvious places where your loved one might hide things. Check the folds of chairs and sofas. Examine handbags or wallets. Look in bowls and dishes in the kitchen.

• If your loved one tends to hoard valuable things, use substitutes. Buy some cheap costume jewellery and store your good stuff in a place your loved one isn't likely to look. If he or she stashes away food that spoils, make packages of savoury biscuits available. Nibbling at various times during the day or night may be the result of legitimate hunger. Provide for this need.

• Keep a 'rummage box' that can be used as a substitute when your loved one starts rummaging through chests or drawers.

• Don't expect your relative to remember the hiding places of the car keys or the post. Asking or demanding will only create a stressful situation. Simply expect to join in the search from time to time.

Rummaging, pillaging, hiding and hoarding are behaviours common to people with dementia. The reasons are unclear, but the need for security may be an underlying factor. Creating a secure environment is a challenge we all face as we care for our loved ones. It is a challenge that can try our patience. It can also make us more tolerant and sensitive people.

Managing Mealtimes

Mealtimes usually include fun and fellowship as well as food. But when you're caring for a person with Alzheimer's, they can be times of frustration.

Eating isn't always a sit-down occasion.

⏮ *My father wouldn't sit down for his meals. He decided he'd rather stand. He'd say, 'I gotta do this' and 'I gotta do that', and then he'd eat a little and run around the house. He was extremely hyperactive. Extremely.*

Judgement and coordination are sometimes affected:

⏮ *My brother can't always judge where his food is. We have to put it in his hand. He does a lot better with finger food, with things he can feel. Cutlery seems too hard for him to manage, and I think he has trouble feeling it because it's so thin. He eats sandwiches, bananas, cheese, things like that.*

The memory for eating and perhaps even for swallowing becomes impaired for some people:

⏮ *My mother sits down at the table but then can't remember how to eat, or what to do with her fork or spoon. I usually have to get her started, and sometimes the old memory seems to come back and kick in. At other times it doesn't, and I have to feed her an entire meal.*

⏮ *It got so it took for ever for my wife to eat. It took over an hour for lunch. Sometimes she'd chew something for ten minutes before she'd swallow it.*

You know how you might stroke a baby's throat sometimes? That's what I'd do with my wife. I'd say, 'Come on, now. Swallow, swallow, swallow.' And then, when she was ready, she'd swallow.

Sometimes a person may refuse to eat. At other times he or she will eat everything in sight.

◄◄ *My husband eats everything he can get his hands on, but he doesn't gain any weight. He runs it off the rest of the time.*

◄◄ *My wife seemed to lose her appetite one day and refused to eat. Now it's a hard job to get anything down her. I know she's depressed, too, and that accounts for some of it.*

People with Alzheimer's, particularly in the later stages, are prone to respiratory infections such as pneumonia. These may be precipitated by choking on food.

◄◄ *Some people with Alzheimer's have trouble swallowing, and instead of food going down their oesophagus it goes down their windpipe. I think that's what happened to my wife. She got pneumonia after an episode of choking one day at the nursing home.*

The following suggestions may help make mealtimes more manageable at various stages in the disease:

• Decrease stimulation in the environment. Maintain a calm atmosphere at mealtimes. Play quiet music instead of loud TV programmes. Consider subdued lighting instead of a bright glare.

• When meal planning, choose from the four basic food groups for a well-rounded diet. These include the following for a day:

Protein. Three servings of the following: lean meats, poultry, fish, cheese, eggs, dried beans, peas, nuts. Egg substitutes and many soy substitutes are also available.

Bread, cereals, starches. Five to seven servings of bread, cereal, rice and other grains. Pasta and potatoes are included in this group. Wholemeal or wholegrain breads are best.

Dairy. Three servings of milk or milk products such as cottage cheese and yoghurt. Fat-free and low-fat milk and milk products are generally recommended and many lactose-free products are available.

Fruits and vegetables. Five to seven servings including dark green or deep yellow vegetables, tomatoes and fruits.[1] Focus on familiar foods your loved one has always liked. Many finger foods, including sandwiches, cheese, fruits and vegetables, can meet the 'basic four' requirements and also meet the needs of a person who is always on the go.

Serving amounts will vary depending on age, height, weight, gender and level of activity. Foods to be avoided are those high in saturated fats and trans fats. Older people may also need some supplements such as vitamin D to assist with calcium absorption. Check with your GP about individual or multiple vitamin supplementation.

• Small, frequent meals or snacks may be more acceptable than large, sit-down dinners three times a day.

• To increase nutrition for the finicky eater, leave snacks around or add the following supplements during the day:
     milk shakes (add ice cream, vanilla, sweetener or flavouring to a glass of milk)
     puddings, custards, yoghurt
     Complan or other dietary supplements

• If swallowing or chewing becomes a problem, try grinding or blending foods. This is preferable to tinned baby foods and enables you to cook the same meal for the whole family. A food processor, blender or small grinder will work well. Thick liquids are often swallowed more easily than thinner liquids. Try cream soups for easier swallowing and added nourishment.

• Try the following steps for alleviating coordination problems:
     Substitute bowls for plates, or consider using a plate guard to minimize accidental spillage.
     Switch to unbreakable dishes.
     Build up utensil handles to make them easier to feel and hold.
     Offer only one food at a time if your loved one has difficulty making choices.

• If you must feed your loved one, consider the following:

Sit, don't stand, when feeding. Maintain eye contact.

Converse naturally, but don't encourage a lot of talking or laughter that could contribute to choking.

Spoons often work better than forks for feeding.

Approach your loved one directly, not from the side. Feed him or her using a gentle, downward pressure on the centre of the tongue.

If there is any weakness or paralysis related to a stroke or vascular dementia, feed on the unaffected side to make chewing and swallowing easier.

Be sensitive to the temperature of foods, especially when foods are microwaved. Your loved one may not be able to communicate discomfort.

Take your time. Don't rush. You may need to encourage your relative to swallow after each bite or make sure food isn't being squirrelled away in ever-bulging cheeks.

• As an added safety precaution, learn the Heimlich or abdominal-thrust manoeuvre. This is a relatively simple procedure that has saved thousands of lives. It involves a series of abdominal thrusts that elevate the diaphragm; air is forced from the lungs by the thrusts to create an artificial cough that can expel an object obstructing the airway. It is something all of us should know, whether or not we have a loved one with Alzheimer's. Hospitals and nursing homes always teach their employees this procedure. You might be able to ask your district nurse to teach you or you could attend a class with St John's Ambulance. If you can't attend a class or demonstration, refer to a first-aid book. See the notes on Chapter Eight for recommended internet websites that include diagrams and more complete explanations of this technique.[2]

• Remember that eating out doesn't have to stop if your loved one has Alzheimer's.

◀◀ *I used to take my wife to a luncheon club run by the community centre in our town. It was good for us both. It got me out and provided her with more stimulation than she had at home. We made a lot of friends there too.*

◄◄ *I take my husband out to eat quite a lot. He sometimes spills things, and occasionally I have to feed him. I have a couple of places that we go to pretty regularly, usually when it's not very crowded. They all know us and the waitresses are great. You don't have to stop doing things you've always enjoyed just because you have Alzheimer's, you know.*

You *don't* have to stop doing things you've always enjoyed. And enjoying a meal with a loved one at home or away from home is one of those things that can still be part of life.

Losing Control

Difficulties with bladder and bowel elimination usually become a problem as Alzheimer's progresses. Incontinence of urine and stool occurs frequently and can present a real physical and emotional dilemma for the unprepared carer. When I was involved in nursing home research I did telephone interviews with carers about primary reasons for placing a relative in a nursing home. I thought that wandering and safety issues might be the primary reasons, but instead, dealing with incontinence appeared to be the most difficult aspect of caring, especially if a loved one needed frequent changing at night. Incontinence can also be embarrassing. It requires us to keep our sense of humour and a sense of perspective.

◄◄ *I remember the day my wife had a bowel movement in the supermarket. I was mortified. But they were so good to us. One young shop assistant came up behind us and rolled up the rug. Luckily my wife did it in the right spot.*

◄◄ *My mother was incontinent once right in the bank. I was cashing a cheque and when I turned around, there she was, taking off her wet pants over by the window. I ran over, grabbed the pants, stuffed them in my handbag, and got her out of there. Fast.*

Just last week I saw a two-year-old in a store downtown do the same thing. Her mother reacted the same way I did. I think you need a sense of humour in this business.

⏮ *My husband is totally incontinent now and has been for quite a while. His urologist told me that one of the things I could expect eventually was lack of control of bowels and bladder. The bad thing about it was that my husband sometimes went to the back of the barn and shed his clothes, including his incontinence pants. He'd throw the wet or soiled pads aside and then put his clothes back on. I think there's quite a pile of those pads out at the back of the barn, in the raspberry bushes.*

In addition to getting rid of our embarrassment, we need to lose the notion that toileting is a very personal, private affair. Sooner or later we'll have to get involved in this aspect of our loved one's care.

⏮ *The biggest problem I had was when my wife first became incontinent. She'd wet the bed at night and I decided, well, I'll just have to get her up. It was tough because she was a sound sleeper and resisted me. Often before I could get her to the toilet she'd urinate on the floor. It used to make me so cross because I didn't understand what was happening.*

Finally I decided there was just no sense trying to get her up and getting angry. It didn't do her any good and it didn't do me any good. So I got some disposable adult nappies, a rubber sheet, and some smaller sheets they call draw sheets, and I put them on the bed. If she was swimming in the morning, that was all right. I just had extra laundry to do.

The following are suggestions for preventing and dealing with incontinence, should it occur, as well as other aspects of bladder and bowel management.

• If incontinence of urine becomes a problem at any stage of Alzheimer's disease, don't assume it's due to the Alzheimer's process. This is especially true if symptoms appear suddenly. There may be an underlying medical problem, such as a urinary-tract infection (UTI). Initially it's wise to talk to your doctor. A simple urine test may be recommended to see if there's an infection that could easily be treated with an antibiotic. Untreated urinary-tract infections can worsen any incontinence related to Alzheimer's.

Women are more prone than men to develop UTIs because it is easier for infectious agents to move up and into the female bladder.

Symptoms of urinary-tract infections and more severe kidney infections can include any or all of the following:

> frequent urge to urinate
> urinating in small amounts
> difficulty starting to urinate
> burning, pain or stinging on urination
> foul-smelling urine
> cloudy, blood-tinged or mucus-containing urine
> abdominal pain or discomfort
> fever and chills
> nausea and vomiting
> back pain
> increased confusion

• Some medications can contribute to urinary incontinence: 'water pills' or diuretics, for example. It's usually best to give these early in the morning to prevent incontinence at night.

Some tranquillizers and sedatives can have the opposite effect and result in urine retention that, if unnoticed and untreated, can be a serious, even life-threatening problem. The medications Haldol or Serenace (haloperidol), frequently prescribed for people with Alzheimer's, are notable examples. Your chemist is usually a good source of information about drug side effects.

If your loved one is on medication that can cause urinary side effects, you need to carefully observe their toileting habits.

• Anticipate accidents. Become aware of mannerisms that may indicate a need to urinate or have a bowel movement.

• Minimize accidents by having a susceptible person cut down on fluid intake, especially tea and coffee, several hours before bedtime.

Fluids should not usually be limited during the day, however, except for other medical reasons. Adequate fluid intake is essential for proper hydration and can also help prevent urinary-tract infections and constipation. If in doubt, check with your doctor. The necessary amount of fluid required for health may vary from person to person. Dehydration as well as overhydration can contribute to confusion.

• Toilet at regular intervals – every two to three hours, before or after meals, and just prior to retiring. Do this even if your loved one wears an incontinence pad or pants. Through regular toileting, a habit pattern can form that may keep him or her dry throughout the day and night. It's definitely worth your effort and a little trial and error. This can also cut down on wandering and agitation.

• Minimize the distance from bedroom to bathroom. Consider the use of a bedside commode.

• Think about using an adult nappy or pad or, for minimal incontinence and dribbling, a sanitary towel or baby's nappy worn inside the underwear. There are many different brands of pants available through chemists and mail order. Costs vary, and it is worth finding out first what is available from the community nursing services. Some people's skin may be sensitive to some makes. You may need to experiment if your relative develops a rash.

Ask your district nurse or Continence Adviser for tips on how to put the adult 'nappies' on when a person is lying down or standing up. Rubber pants are also available in adult sizes.

Protective pads may help your loved one (and you) feel more secure when out and about, though there is often an understandable initial reaction to 'needing to wear nappies again, like a baby', as one carer put it. If your relative does not take them off at night, incontinence pads may help you both get a good night's rest. Be sensitive, though, to your loved one's feelings of shame, embarrassment and loss of self-esteem.

• Skin tissue is very sensitive to urine and can break down quickly if not kept clean and dry. Soap and water is generally all you need. Avoid perfumed or scented powders: they can contribute to urinary-tract infections. If perspiration around skin folds in the abdomen and groin area is a problem, talc powders and talc-free powders are available. Cornflour is another alternative but people with corn allergies can also have allergic reactions to this powder. Check with a chemist about alternative products if there are any signs of an allergic skin reaction. Your GP may also order a medicated cream and some types are available without prescription to alleviate skin irritation.

As with urine, stool on the skin can result in skin breakdown and even urinary-tract infections. If you need to assist your loved one with hygiene, wipe and wash well, wiping and/or washing from front (urinary opening) to back (rectal area).

• Protect the bed with a waterproof mattress cover. A large sheet of plastic or an old shower curtain also works well. Disposable or cloth bed pads with waterproof backing are available and can cut down on laundry. Simple draw sheets (smaller pieces of sheeting) or pillowcases with a piece of plastic inside may also work well and are inexpensive alternatives.

To control odours from urine, wash mattress covers regularly with soap and water, and spray with a disinfectant.

Some areas have an incontinence laundry service which can be a great help for carers. It is worth asking your district nurse whether such a service is available.

• Indwelling catheters are usually not recommended for the management of incontinence because they can easily contribute to infections and are often pulled out by people with dementia.

External catheters that fit like condoms may, however, be useful for some men who experience incontinence at night and are heavy sleepers.

• If urinary retention and difficulty starting a urine stream are problems, try running water in the sink or bath when your loved one is on the toilet. Your GP should be able to provide information on how to contact a local Continence Adviser for further help.

• Bowel habits differ from person to person. Some people move their bowels daily, others every two to three days. A person with dementia may have difficulty keeping a normal schedule for a variety of reasons related to the disease process: diet, lack of exercise, various medications, and so on. If diarrhoea is a problem, it may be related to a stomach upset or injudicious use of laxatives.

A more frequently occurring problem is constipation. Signs of constipation include pain in the abdominal or rectal area, irregular and infrequent bowel movements, discomfort or pain when having a bowel movement, diarrhoea or liquid leakage around a hard, impacted stool, and headache.

The best way to prevent constipation is through a diet adequate in liquids, fibre and bulk. Breakfast is often the best meal for adding fibre. You might try sprinkling bran on hot cereal or serving a high fibre cereal. (A fibre cereal mixed with yoghurt and fruit is a nutritious way to increase fibre and bulk.) Substitute wholemeal breads for white. Generally add more raw fruits and vegetables to the menu of the person you care for unless some other medical problem exists that requires a low fibre diet.

• Lack of exercise can contribute to constipation. Remember the therapeutic value of walking.

• Constipation is also a frequent side effect of some medications, especially those prescribed for pain. Ask your chemist. You may need to switch to another type of pain reliever if the problem persists.

If diet and exercise fail to work, consider the use of stool softeners, either prescription or over-the-counter. Some are available in liquid or powder form. Overuse of laxatives such as milk of magnesia may lead to bowel inactivity. Avoid them, if possible.

• Suppositories may help some people. They are available in mild over-the-counter forms or by prescription. Chemists also carry various name-brand and generic-brand enemas that are relatively easy to administer and may need to be used on occasion. If you have any questions about how to give an enema, check with your district nurse.

Losing control can be an embarrassment for the Alzheimer's sufferer and a management problem for the carer. But we need to remember that it is a *manageable* problem, a problem that can be minimized with the proper resources and our resourcefulness.

Sexual Disinhibitions

◄◄ *My husband undresses himself a lot in the nursing home, right in the middle of the dining room. Sometimes he asks the other residents and even the aides if they will go to bed with him. If he were in his right mind he'd be humiliated.*

◄◄ *My sister was always a very shy, withdrawn person but she isn't any more. You should hear the language that comes out of her mouth when they try to give her a shower. She also tries to grab people if they get too close to her – and not in very acceptable places.*

Loss of impulse control, causing a person to engage in inappropriate sexual behaviour of which they are not aware because of their state of disorientation, is not common to most Alzheimer's sufferers. But when it does occur it can be particularly distressing to the family carer at home. If their loved one is in a nursing care facility, family members need to know their loved one will be treated with dignity and respect and not made fun of or be treated with contempt.

Often behaviour that may appear sexual in nature may be caused by various other factors. For example, the person who wanders around partially clothed or with a blouse unbuttoned or trousers unzipped may have simply forgotten how to dress themselves. Due to the degree of their dementia, they may be totally unaware of their state of undress.

A calm, gentle but firm approach to reorient a person back to their bedroom or a bathroom where you can assist them in re-dressing is often all that is needed to solve the problem. In nursing homes, trying to re-dress a person in a busy hall or a noisy dining area will often precipitate a catastrophic reaction. The person may think they are being molested; not a few persons with Alzheimer's have cried 'rape' when carers with good intentions have tried to help them.

If zippers on trousers are continually becoming unzipped and shirts and blouses unbuttoned, switch to pull-on trousers and pull-over shirts and sweaters. Dresses that zip up at the back are better for women who have a tendency to fidget with their clothes.

Masturbation may also occur in public places and may be engaged in simply because it feels good to the brain-damaged person. Distraction will often work if the person's attention can be redirected to something else to hold or touch. Masturbation can also be prompted by poor genital hygiene, or itching related to a urinary-tract infection that prompts rubbing the genital area for relief. Carefully assess possible underlying physical reasons for this behaviour, such as the adequacy of hygiene.

Sexual overtures, or what are interpreted as sexual overtures, may be made in nursing home or hospital settings to other residents, patients, visitors and staff members. Often the person with dementia will simply mistake the other person for a beloved spouse and treat them accordingly. They may climb into bed with another resident of the opposite sex, simply because they have always slept with a spouse and have no idea that this is not their own room or their own bed. A gentle but firm approach can guide the person with dementia back to their own room and bed; the rights of other residents need to be protected, but the affectional needs for closeness and companionship of the person with dementia should also be addressed.

The impact of Alzheimer's on the marital relationship, including all the varying dimensions of sexuality and intimacy, can be devastating for carers. As Lore Wright notes in *Alzheimer's Disease and Marriage*, Robert Browning's poem that includes the familiar lines, 'Grow old along with me! The best is yet to be…' rings hollow for many couples when a spouse has Alzheimer's.[3]

Sensitive marital counselling with a professional who is very familiar with Alzheimer's disease may be needed. Other spouses who are carers can also be supportive and may welcome the opportunity to share concerns and strategies with others in similar situations.

Chapter Nine

The Struggle for Safety

Safety is always an issue for older people, especially those living alone and in frail health. Add dementia, and safety becomes an all-consuming concern that can spell disaster. Preventive measures have to be taken. And, fortunately, there are many things we can do to ensure our loved one's safety, as well as our own.

Taking Away the Car Keys

Most of us drive by habit. If the way is familiar, we're often unaware of the various roads we pass or the towns we drive through. Yet if the sudden and unexpected should occur, all our senses go on the alert. We are usually able to make a quick judgement, respond appropriately and avoid an accident.

This may not be the case, though, for Alzheimer's sufferers, who may be unable to respond quickly or logically to a sudden, unexpected event. Research comparing persons diagnosed with Alzheimer's to older adults without symptoms of dementia indicates that persons with dementia show statistically significant differences in their ability to react to dangerous situations commonly encountered when driving, as well as differences in ability to execute emergency measures to avoid accidents. Although vision may remain intact and hearing may be unaffected, the ability to make decisions about what they are seeing and hearing – and even where they are going – is progressively impaired.

⏮ *One day my husband turned around, right in the middle of the road. We were on the main street in the city at the time. The next thing I knew, we were headed up the slip road – going the wrong way – on the motorway.*

I said to myself, 'This is it. I can't cope with this any longer.'

◄◄ *I used to pray every day for other drivers because my father was a maniac on the road. He had been an excellent mechanic and driver, but as his disease progressed he became careless and dangerous. He gave me a ride one day that was enough to make my hair turn white. It was the most awful experience of my life.*

Our identity is partly defined for us by the things we do, particularly the things we do well. Driving is something most of us, especially men, are expected to do and to do well.

Being told you cannot drive, that you are no longer safe on the road, can be a tremendous blow to a person's ego. Regardless of the degree of memory impairment, a person still responds on a feeling level when identity is threatened. People with Alzheimer's often won't relinquish the wheel voluntarily.

◄◄ *My husband's driving drove me crazy, but I couldn't convince him to stop. You'd think he'd been on a ten-day drinking binge the way he acted behind the wheel.*

I'd shout, I'd scream, I'd stamp my feet. I even threatened to leave him once. It didn't make any difference. He kept insisting he could drive just fine.

◄◄ *My car was being fixed the day we had our family reunion. After the reunion Dad took me to the garage and he started following a motorcycle driver. He was only about two feet ahead of us and the poor guy couldn't go any faster. He was behind another car, sandwiched in by my father.*

I said, 'Don't you think you're a little close?'

He just glared at me and said, 'Oh, it's all right.' He could never understand that his judgement was wrong.

Convincing a loved one to stop driving may be the most difficult thing we'll ever have to do as carers. But it must be done; usually the sooner, the better.

How soon is *soon*? We can take our cues from our loved one. A diagnosis of dementia alone is not a reason to stop driving, but many symptoms associated with advancing dementia *are* valid reasons. If there are obvious impairments in other areas of their behaviour that involve judgement, concentration and coordination, as well as time, place and person orientation, the ability to drive safely will also be impaired. And it will only worsen.[1]

The following strategies may be helpful:

• Begin with a gentle person-to-person approach. You may find yourself pleasantly surprised. Your loved one may consider it a relief not to have to drive. Don't assume he or she wants to continue driving.

• Many carers find that it helps to pray before talking with the loved one. Avoid judging or criticizing driving skills. Instead, consider the person's feelings and empathize. It should be easy: you know how you'd feel if you were in a similar position. Focus on the safety issues involved.

• One carer told me, 'I hid my husband's glasses. I hid the car keys. I removed the distributor cap. I disconnected the starter wire. Alzheimer's makes you real sneaky.'

You may have to do any or all of these things at some point if your loved one insists on driving, though perhaps a better solution is to visibly remove the object of the temptation. If you don't drive, this shouldn't be a problem. If you do, check with a neighbour or a nearby garage about keeping your vehicle for your use only.

• Ask your GP to speak with your loved one or write a letter or a 'prescription' stating he or she can no longer drive.

⏮ *The doctor helped me out and it worked just fine. He took my husband into his surgery, sat him down and said, 'George, how many years have you been driving? Don't you think it would be a good idea if you sat in the passenger seat for a while and let your wife do the driving for you both?'*

I guess it must have been the voice of authority. I never had to speak about it to my husband again. He just stopped driving.

◄◄ *My father was always a respecter of the law regarding his driving licence. He knew you couldn't get into the car without it. He would always say, 'Have I got my licence?'*

We finally convinced the doctor that Dad was dangerous on the road. The doctor wrote him a letter stating he could no longer drive. When we got the letter, my dad gave my mother his licence. He just voluntarily handed it over. He seemed to respect the doctor's authority.

Someone else may have the voice of authority in your loved one's life – your doctor, the insurance company, a solicitor or the Department of Transport. If this is the case, enlist their help. Stress the importance of safety for both your loved one and other people.

The Driver and Vehicle Licensing Agency (DVLA) deals confidentially with enquiries about disabilities affecting a person's fitness to drive. Anyone who holds a current driving licence or wants to reapply for a new licence and has a medical condition such as dementia that could affect their driving judgement and ability, currently or in the future, must provide information about their health status to the DVLA; failure to notify the agency is a criminal offence. The DVLA will contact the person's physician for more information; if the person is allowed to drive, the DVLA will request periodic reports from the person's GP. Physicians can also contact the DVLA directly if they think a patient diagnosed with dementia has failed to notify the agency. The person's insurance company should also be notified immediately. (See Appendix D for DVLA website information.) If your loved one lives alone but still has a desire to get out and about, you'll need to provide transportation that is safe. Sharing the responsibility with family members, friends and neighbours can ease the burden. Taxi services or a bus pass may be an economical alternative in some areas. Both people with Alzheimer's and carers should qualify for half-priced disabled travel on British Rail and London Underground. Enquire about transportation options through your local Social Services or through community organizations that serve the elderly. Regular routes that transport people to and from day centres, for example, might help meet your loved one's need for socialization and nutrition, as well as the need to be 'on the go'.

If you hire home-care workers and feel it is safe for your loved one to ride in a car, consider employing at least one aide who is willing to drive and is appropriately licensed and insured. If you hire through an agency, check its transportation policies. Some agencies will not allow employees to transport others but may forget to tell you this when you apply for help.

You may never have thought of yourself as adventurous. A spouse with Alzheimer's may change all that, particularly if getting out and about is important to you. If you don't drive and want to learn, find out about taking lessons. Learning to drive at the age of fifty-five or sixty is not impossible or impractical. In fact, it may be the best gift you can give yourself both now and for the future.

Finally, 'treat' your loved one. Say, 'It's time you relaxed and enjoyed the view,' as one carer successfully told her husband. You may discover that you will both actually enjoy yourselves and the scenery for the first time in months.

Remember, driving is one learned activity that quickly becomes unlearned. It's therefore a dangerous activity for someone with Alzheimer's. Driving is also a habit. Like most habits, if it's not practised, it soon fades away. It's important that it fades before any serious or tragic injuries occur.

Home Safety

Safety in and around the house is always a concern for the older person, especially the older person who lives alone. Add any degree of confusion and disorientation and the potential for disaster is multiplied.

◄◄ *We no longer wanted to leave my mother alone, not even for a little while. We were always afraid she'd start a fire with her smoking. She'd light the wrong end of the cigarette sometimes and try to put it in her mouth. She'd also drop*

---

cigarettes when they were lit or stuff them in the corners of the couch to put them out. She had a plastic tablecloth on the kitchen table that was covered with cigarette burns.

◄◄ We had a pile of wood in the garage, and one day we found my father trying to light it with a blow torch. We took the torch away. Anything we thought might be dangerous we took away.

One day we found Dad turning on the flame on the gas cooker. You know those inspection lights you use, the ones at the end of a long cord? Well, we'd bought one, a good one, and Dad had it. He'd cut it all up into pieces and was trying to weld it together again with the flames of the cooker.

When I tried to take it away from him, he shouted at me for buying something 'cheap and inferior'. He told me it was no good.

All I can say is, you have to be alert!

What is a safety hazard for one person may not be a hazard for another. An iron may present no problem to a man who has never ironed in his life, and an older woman may not feel the urge to rummage through her husband's tool-box.

We don't have to totally reconstruct our houses, but we do have to know our loved one's habits. We have to be alert. Decide what are potential hazards for your loved one, remembering that these may change as the disease progresses. Here are some specific situations to consider:

1. Prevent burns from fire, water and electricity

• Lock up electrical equipment such as hair dryers and electric shavers if there is danger your loved one may plug them in and drop them in the sink or bath.

• Turn down the temperature of your water heater if your loved one can no longer judge hot from cold.

• Monitor smoking by keeping matches and lighters in your possession. Many carers have found that breaking a lifelong habit of smoking is unexpectedly easy for someone with Alzheimer's. Cigarettes, cigars and pipes that are out of sight may quickly fade out of mind as well.

• Remove knobs from your gas cooker or turn off the shut-off valve at night if your loved one wanders and tries to cook.

• Unplug electrical appliances in the kitchen. Consider coverings for electrical outlets.

• Have a fire extinguisher in your kitchen that can be used for all types of fire. Install smoke detectors in appropriate places and test them regularly.

• Plan escape routes from the various rooms in your house in case there is ever a need to evacuate.

2. Minimize cuts and bruises

• Lock up knives, power tools and other sharp objects.

• Pad the corners of sharp pieces of furniture.

• Check glassware and other dishes periodically for cracks.

3. Avoid accidental poisoning

• Keep medications in a safe, dry place, not in a kitchen cabinet or the bathroom medicine chest. If necessary, lock them up.

• Lock up poisonous cleaning supplies or store them in inaccessible places.

• Be aware of the signs of poisoning, which may include any of the following:
    nausea, vomiting, diarrhoea
    severe abdominal pain, cramping
    slow breathing and slow pulse

profuse sweating or salivation

obvious burns or stains around the mouth

odours on the breath, such as paraffin or turpentine

unconsciousness

convulsions

• If you do need to go to the hospital, remember to take any empty bottles or containers with you to show what has been swallowed.

4. Decrease the danger of falls

Falls become more problematic as Alzheimer's disease progresses and areas of the brain that control muscles and coordination are affected.

The following tips can help accident-proof your home against falls.

• Avoid high-gloss waxing of vinyl or wood floors.

• Eliminate loose rugs or anchor them firmly, especially in the bathroom.

• Make sure all electrical and phone cords are outside high-traffic areas.

• Get rid of chairs that tip over easily. Solid and familiar furniture, strategically placed, can be an ambulation aid.

• Clear away clutter, especially on stairs.

• Remove raised doorway thresholds and replace them with flat, flush stripping.

• Put locks at the top or bottom of cellar and exit doors. Lock windows if necessary or disguise them with curtains. Alarms can also be installed on windows and doors.

• Store frequently used items in easily reached places.

• Light up nocturnal trips from bedroom to toilet with a 25-watt soft-light bulb, or consider night-lights in various rooms.

• Install safety rails in areas around toilet, bath and shower. Use suction mats or non-slip bath mats in bath and shower.

• Periodically check the soles and heels of shoes and slippers for wear. Thin, worn soles can be slippery.

• Avoid long hems and trailing sleeves in your loved one's nightwear.

• Falls most frequently occur on the top or bottom step. Paint both steps in contrasting colours or use bright paint strips.

• Make sure stair rails are solid and secure.

• Block the bottom and top of the stairs with a sturdy gate if needed.

• Outside, make sure your driveway is well lit, pond or pool areas are well secured, and pavements are in good repair.

• If your loved one needs help walking, consider purchasing a stick or a Zimmer walking frame. Zimmer frames are generally made from aluminium and have four feet fitted with rubber grips; some are foldable, making them easier to fit into a car. Another possibility is a walking belt. (This can also be used to help get a person in and out of a chair or bed with minimal effort on the part of the carer.) Ask the physiotherapist or district nurse for a demonstration.

• Various types of alarm can be worn by people with dementia to summon help in case they fall and can't reach the phone. Movement detectors can also be installed to allow a third party to monitor movement around a home; via the internet, movement can be monitored if the person leaves the home. This can be helpful for fall monitoring but also for wandering off.

Finally, if your loved one should fall, don't panic. Be especially careful if you attempt to break the fall. Take time to assess the situation. It may be an emergency, but chances are it is not life-threatening.

If for any reason you suspect a fracture or head injury, *do not attempt to move your loved one*. Simply make him or her as comfortable as possible. Use a blanket to prevent chilling, and use a rolled-up blanket or pillow to support an injured limb. Then call the ambulance for help. Don't ask friends or neighbours to help you move your loved one to a more comfortable position; this could cause further damage to a fractured limb.

Some signs of a fracture include:

• pain or tenderness in the injured area that increases with pressure or movement

• deformity (for example, a fractured hip may cause one leg to appear shorter and to rotate outward)

• swelling (not always immediate)

• discolouration or bruising

• exposed bone ends that have broken through the skin

• possible shock (cold, pale, clammy skin; rapid pulse; shallow breathing)

If you don't suspect a fracture, but are not sure you can help your loved one on your own, get help. Call a neighbour or the police.

Falling can be a symptom of other problems, such as medication side effects, poor vision, small strokes, low blood pressure and so on. A physical examination may be in order if you notice any obvious and sudden changes in your loved one's ability to navigate around the house.

Educate Yourself and Be Prepared

Investing in a good first-aid manual can help you feel more confident if an emergency should arise. You might also want to purchase a first-aid kit or have the following supplies on hand:

• adhesive plasters

• large and small sterile gauze dressings

• crêpe bandages

- surgical adhesive tape

- scissors and safety pins

- a triangular bandage

- an eye bath

- ice packs you can keep in the freezer

Home safety for the person with Alzheimer's is much the same as home safety for anyone else: a little common sense, a little foresight into possible hazards, and a little knowledge of what to do and when to do it goes a long way.

When the Emergency is You

'In the event of an emergency,' I told one of the agency helpers I'd hired, 'I can be reached at my work phone number.'

'Fine,' she said. 'But what if the emergency is *you*? What if you get hit by a bus or your car lands in a ditch? What do I do with your mother?

I had never really thought about it.

As carers for people with Alzheimer's, we hope and pray *we* won't ever end up as a medical or surgical emergency, but that possibility is always present. Contrary to what most of us would like to believe, we're not immune from our own disasters, or even death.

There's a good motto for carers who find themselves thinking about their own mortality: Be prepared.

Emergency numbers

If aides care for your loved one in your home while you are away, the substitute carers should know how to reach you. Provide them with a list of emergency phone numbers that might include:

- relative(s), friend(s), neighbour(s)

- your GP; your relative's GP

- the hospital accident and emergency department

Substitute carers need to know who will be responsible for your loved one should you suddenly become incapacitated. Who, specifically, should they call? They should also have the Social Services number in case no one on their list can be contacted and emergency caring arrangements need to be made.

Keep a list of emergency numbers at home even if you don't hire help. It will be available in times of need.

If your loved one stays at a day-care centre, you will need to tell the staff where you can be reached and provide information about what to do if something should happen to you.

Prepare emergency-care notebooks

Some carers keep a notebook of all the vital information someone else would need in order to assume caring responsibilities in case of an emergency.

Setting aside a few hours to organize such a notebook will be well worth the effort and can contribute to your peace of mind. A notebook will prove an invaluable resource if a substitute carer comes into your home to look after your relative. It can also benefit carers in a residential home or nursing home setting if your loved one needs alternative living arrangements. Your notebook might include some of the following information:

• *Daily routine.* If the person you care for has a daily routine, it's wise to include this in as much detail as possible. For example, '7:00 – Usually wakes up. 7:15 – Help out of bed to bedside commode. 7:30 – Give sponge bath and dress.' What can your loved one do independently? What do you have to help with?

• *Nutritional needs.* What are your relative's eating habits and problems? Are there favourite foods? Dislikes? Allergies? Is there a favourite area to eat in? Any special dishes or utensils? Can your relative feed himself or herself? Does he or she snack during the day?

• *Sleep patterns.* What is the normal bedtime routine? Are naps common? If night-time wandering is a problem, what do you do to manage this behaviour?

• *Toileting concerns.* If there's a special toileting routine to prevent or control incontinence, include details for both bladder and bowel habits.

• *Medications.* What medications are taken? Include the name of each drug, dosage and time to be taken. Does the person you care for swallow pills without difficulty, or do pills have to be crushed and given in food or drink?

• *Special behaviour problems.* If there are any specific problems, such as wandering or 'sundowning', include these. (See pp. 97–112 for additional examples.)

• *Social history.* Jot down anything that will make communication with your relative easier – the name he or she likes to be called, information about likes, dislikes, interests, occupation. Help the substitute carer know your loved one as a person to relate to, not a problem to solve.

Watching Over Your Loved One

It is impossible to prepare for every calamity that might occur in our lives as carers. But several additional safety measures can provide important safeguards against the unknown.

For example, if your own health is frail, consider installing an emergency-response unit at home that can be attached to your telephone. Commonly known as 'life-lines', these units can be activated at the press of a button (usually carried or worn). Some local councils provide them free for elderly and infirm people.

Identification jewellery can be especially vital for your loved one should the two of you be involved in an accident or should you suddenly become ill.

If you suddenly need to go to the hospital and there is no time to make emergency arrangements, insist that your loved one go with you. Have the hospital social worker notified en route or upon arrival so that special arrangements can be made for his or her care. Carry emergency numbers with you in a wallet or purse.

It is sometimes wise planning to arrange for someone to have power of attorney over you as well as over your loved one, in case you become incapacitated. Talk with your solicitor or Citizens' Advice Bureau about this. You may also wish to appoint someone else as an authorized agent to collect pensions and benefits from the Post Office, if you find it difficult to get out.

It's never pleasant to think about our own ill health, but denial of the possibility is guaranteed to bring future grief should we suddenly become dependent.

Plan ahead. Be prepared.

PART THREE

Caring for Yourself

The deepest lessons come out of the
deepest waters and the hottest fires.

ELISABETH ELLIOT, *A PATH*
THROUGH SUFFERING

Chapter Ten

People Who Help

I have always thought of myself as an active person. My solo lifestyle for many years meant a full-time job plus numerous activities outside the home. Moving back home to care for two older parents with health problems (my father was diagnosed with cancer) threatened to change all that.

When it came to affording expensive private care, my parents and I were not very wealthy. Our collective income was not low enough to make us eligible for any supplementary health programmes offered in the United States and not high enough to afford many services either. Also, many services available in more metropolitan areas were simply not available in our predominantly rural area. I quickly realized that creative and cost-effective measures were in order if I wanted to maintain my own emotional and physical health. Caring can take its toll on both. If I wanted to continue to work full-time or even part-time, I knew I was going to need additional resources and resource people.

A verse in the Bible begins, 'Carry each other's burdens' (Galatians 6:2). There are many burdens we can help each other carry. As carers, we need other people to help us. We need to learn to lean. We also need to know who to lean on, who to call on for help.

Leaning on others is not a sign of weakness. Admitting we need other people to help us occasionally can be a sign of strength – as well as a great relief. Allowing others to help us strengthens us for our caring responsibilities.

Help can come in many forms and from a surprising number of places. Specific services will vary, depending on which country and which part of your country you live in, but there are many available. This section looks at a variety of support systems available to the carer and offers some suggestions for using them. Caring is hard, but it doesn't have to be an unbearable burden. There are many ways to lighten the load.

Support Groups

My mother wandered, never slept at night, and repeated the same words and phrases dozens of times a day. But it was my father who needed help most. Mother was well taken care of, but my dad suffered from frayed emotions, fatigue and a flagging spirit.

Dad needed a support group. And when I moved back home to help him care for my mother, I found that I needed one too.

Shortly after I returned home, a letter in our newspaper gave the phone number for a local Alzheimer's support group. I called the number and talked with one of the support group members for over an hour. She invited me to a meeting and encouraged me to take Mum to a doctor who was willing to do a complete physical, including a variety of blood tests and a CAT scan. She said we'd both be better able to cope if we knew what we were dealing with and could share our concerns with others.

She was right.

Local organized support or self-help groups are scattered all over the country wherever family members provide care. They meet in homes, hospitals, nursing homes and churches. They come in all shapes and sizes, adapting themselves to the various needs represented by group members. Some are formal, with well-structured programmes. Others are informal discussions. Some are a combination of the two. Regardless of their structure, support groups are made up of other people who can prop you up when you are weary.

When I called the local support group, I discovered that Dad and I weren't alone. There were many other people in our county, some even in our own neighbourhood, who really understood our situation. They were *in* our situation.

◄◄ *Sometimes you feel like you're the only person in the world with a family situation like yours. And then you go to a support group meeting and you realize there are other people very much like you.*

◄◄ *Sometimes I get very lonely. I have friends, but they're not the same as the friends I've made through the support group. I find I need both.*

Support groups can contribute to our own emotional and spiritual well-being:

◄◄ *After a while you begin to wonder if you're seeing things in their proper perspective. You feel like you're dealing with something all by yourself. But when you're able to talk with other people and listen to their experiences, you realize you're still okay yourself. You're not going off the deep end.*

◄◄ *The support group was a place where I could share my real feelings. Even the negative ones – my guilt and my pain. No one ever said, 'You shouldn't feel that way,' because they all knew exactly what I was feeling. And why.*

Support groups can offer us more than just a listening ear. Often their help comes in very practical, material ways:

◄◄ *The generosity of the support group overwhelmed me. They raised the money for our travel and the overnight stay in a motel when I had to take my husband to a research centre to be involved in an experimental drug trial.*

◄◄ *We laugh a lot in our support group. Not at our loved ones, but at some of the things they do. Many things are funny, though not at the time, when we're usually angry and frustrated. But after it's all over we need to be able to share. And to laugh. You can't do that with everyone. Some people would get offended and would think we have some sick sense of humour. But most of us realize laughter is therapy.*

Support groups can even help with difficult decisions, such as whether to institutionalize our loved one or request a post-mortem.

⏮ *The support group guided me to a special psychiatric hospital where my husband is now. One support group member, who knew I couldn't face the fact that my husband needed institutionalization, said to me, 'Have you considered the psychiatric hospital? My wife has been there for ten years and she has received excellent care. Don't let preconceptions about "mental institutions" prevent you from looking into it.'*

I called that hospital. I never would have done that without encouragement. It's a great place.

⏮ *Through the support group I first heard about the need for post-mortems and how to make arrangements. The group helped me sort through my feelings and make a decision.*

Support groups are not only for carers whose loved ones are still living. Many groups include surviving spouses and relatives. Their reasons for continued involvement are varied.

⏮ *My wife died four years ago and I still go to the support group. I feel that, having gone through all this, maybe I can help someone else. I think that's the way all of us who have lost spouses or parents feel. Our trials are over, but maybe we can help someone whose trials aren't.*

⏮ *The support group fulfils a need in me to help other people. I hope that the little I can share can help relieve the problems of others.*

Support groups aren't just for people who care for loved ones at home. Many carers whose loved ones are in nursing homes or hospitals continue to attend meetings.

⏮ *There are a lot of people who come to our support group who have relatives in nursing homes. Sometimes visiting loved* ones in a nursing home is harder than if they were at home with you. It's a different kind of hard. We still need support.

◄◄ *The group I belong to actually meets in the nursing home where my mother is staying. It's great. The social worker leads it and we have the opportunity to ask questions. They bring in different speakers and we learn a lot. It's a nice group of people.*

Support groups aren't something you should feel obliged to join. There may be a wrong time or a right time to take part:

◄◄ *My first experience at a local group meeting was traumatic. I didn't want to hear about what might happen to my husband. He wasn't that bad yet, and I couldn't face the thought that he might be tied to a chair all day, playing with his shoelaces. He was still driving at the time and I didn't want to hear how bad it was going to be. I went to the group once and then came back, a year later. Then I was ready to hear.*

◄◄ *I'm a very private person. I just can't share my feelings in a group. I went once and felt uncomfortable. But I do keep in touch with several of the support group members. That helps a lot.*

Groups can be helpful even if you don't think you'd be comfortable voicing your concerns in front of others, or if you simply can't get out because of caring responsibilities.

◄◄ *I wasn't able to get out to the support group for two years; I didn't have anyone to care for my wife. So the group came individually and visited me. I will always be grateful.*

As these carers have mentioned, most support groups have members who are willing to talk on the telephone, send information or channel you to appropriate resources and literature. They can also offer suggestions on management issues and other carer concerns, such as finances and nursing home placement. And sometimes group members do make home visits to encourage carers who cannot come to meetings.

To find out about support groups in your area, contact the Alzheimer's Society or a local Age Concern office. They can help you start a support group if there are none in your area.

Support groups aren't just for adults. They can also include teenagers. If there are a number of carers with teens, consider establishing a separate group for the young people. If guidance is needed, it may be available through a group member or someone else in the community, such as a minister, psychologist, psychotherapist or counsellor. You could also ask for help from Youth Access (see Appendix D for this address). Bringing teens and parents together for an informal picnic or potluck lunch might be a good place to start. *Helping Children and Teens Understand Alzheimer's Disease*, for example, is a helpful brochure available from the Alzheimer's Association in the United States and is available online.[1]

Lastly, support groups can help you feel more in control of what seems to be an uncontrollable situation. They can help you get actively engaged in the battle against Alzheimer's in a variety of ways.

◄◄ *Our local group does a lot in the community. We sponsor workshops, supply speakers for churches and service clubs, distribute literature at health fairs and even our county fair. We help educate the community and increase awareness.*

◄◄ *Through the support group I learned how to be more involved politically, and how I could take my experience of pain and make a small difference in the world. I've written letters to politicians about the financial needs of Alzheimer's families. Then I went to some meetings of the community health council. One of these days I might even have the courage to speak more publicly about it.*

A motto coined by the Alzheimer's Association in the United States in the late 1980s was 'Someone to stand by you'. The motto for local support groups could well be 'Someone to walk with you'. That is what Alzheimer's support groups have to offer.

Friends and Relations

Some carers report that their circle of friends has become more restricted as a result of their loved one's illness. Others have discovered many new friendships. One thing is certain for all: if it weren't for friends to confide in, caring would be a very lonely business.

> ◄◄ *I have a wonderful friend I can go to at any time. It started three years ago when she fell and broke her hip. After she came home from the hospital, I went every day and helped her put on her shoes and stockings. Sometimes I'd go early in the morning before my husband got out of bed. Other times I'd take him with me. I'd wash her feet, maybe cut her toenails, and we'd talk. She told me once, 'I want to pay you for helping me.' And I said to her, 'Are you crazy? Don't you know how much a good psychiatrist costs? I should be paying you!' She is wonderful. She simply listens.*

Neighbours and relatives can also be helpful when we need a short break in the day's care.

> ◄◄ *I had a neighbour who was very good to us. I'd take my wife over once a week and she'd just sit and watch TV. She was no trouble at all, the neighbour said. No trouble at all.*

> ◄◄ *Our neighbour always had an open door, which was good because my mother wandered through it a lot! The neighbour sat her down, got her a cup of coffee and called us to say my mother was there and all right.*

> ◄◄ *My daughter-in-law's a hairdresser. Every Saturday she does my wife's hair at her house, which is not the easiest thing to do, because my wife gets up about five or six times and wanders around. That's my free time. It's the only chance I get during the week to mow the lawn or to talk on the phone without getting interrupted.*

Sometimes friends and neighbours may avoid us. Often this happens because of their own emotional response to Alzheimer's disease, not because of an uncaring attitude or rudeness.

Visits from a person with Alzheimer's may remind our friends and neighbours of their own advancing age and mortality, two things many people would like to forget. Reasons for what carers perceive to be fair-weather friends or neglectful neighbours vary.

⏪ *I really wanted to visit, but I didn't do it very much. I know my best friend's wife thought it was a lack of caring on my part. It wasn't. I was just plain scared. Now that he's dead I feel guilty. What can I say?*

The same may be true of relatives who you may feel have abandoned your sinking ship and are shirking their responsibilities. Carers often express feelings of anger, resentment and frustration because of perceived abandonment. However, relatives may simply be unable to face their own fears and their loved one's failing health and frailty.

⏪ *You should have seen my wife's brother. He was furious when he found out she was in a nursing home. When he finally went up and saw her, she didn't know him. He said to me, 'I didn't know she was this bad.' I said, 'I've been trying to tell you for three years, but you wouldn't believe me.' Later he told me he didn't want to believe it.*

⏪ *It bothers me that my oldest child hasn't been to see his grandmother in over three years. But he can't seem to take it. He gets emotional when he's there and he starts to cry. And he's thirty-eight years old. On one hand, I think he should make himself go. But then, I suppose, she doesn't know him anyway. Maybe it doesn't matter.*

⏪ *In our case it's been much harder for the two oldest siblings to visit. They can't face it. In a dire emergency they might be of help, but not now, not on a steady basis. They're dealing with their own concerns about their future and also their own hurt and pain in facing the current situation. I know it's very painful. I hurt too. It's especially hard on my father and mother.*

◄◄ My brother lives in another state and, when he calls, he never talks about Dad. He keeps it inside.

One day he did visit, and he went with us to the nursing home. He didn't want to go, but I said to him, 'You've been away for several years and you have no idea what's going on. I think it would be a good idea if you went out to see Dad. In fact, maybe you think it's a lot more gruesome than it actually is.'

So my brother went with us and we sat and talked to Dad, or, rather, my mother and I sat and talked to Dad. I don't think my brother could understand how we could be so cool about it. We talked and laughed and fed Dad lunch while the kids were in the background, banging on the piano. My brother sat and watched us and didn't say a word. At one point I said, 'Are you glad you came?' and he said, 'Yes,' and that was the end of that.

It's sad because I think my brother has been dying inside all these years. His best friend says he won't talk about it to him either. Maybe he's handling it. I hope so.

We'd all like to think that a chronic illness such as Alzheimer's would bring families and friends closer together, not pull them apart. It can do both, depending to some extent on our attitude as carers and our willingness to understand and help our other loved ones. We may, at times, have to be gentle and forgiving in the midst of our own emotional upheavals. Life is too short and relationships are too valuable to carry grudges.

Yet sometimes the problem isn't a difficulty in dealing with emotions at all. Not everyone is comfortable being a carer or being around people who are physically or mentally impaired. Families and friends may not know what they can do. They may feel awkward. Or they may want to help but fear they'll be invading our privacy. Sometimes they need us to give them permission to help us. We can do this by asking them for assistance or advice.

There are many ways that friends and relations can offer support to their loved one and to the primary caregiver. One carer told me how her whole family gets involved in their mother's care, even though they are separated by distance. Geography doesn't seem to be a barrier for this family. Though distance precludes day-to-day care, they make periodic visits and work together as a team.

The son is the problem solver. He uses his expertise to help with financial and legal problems. One sister is the organizer. She helped get her parents Meals-on-Wheels and a place at the day centre, and she organized information about an experimental drug programme her mother became involved with.

Another is the practical manager. She takes her mother shopping when she visits, alters clothing and takes home special laundry, helping in practical ways.

A third sister is the sounding board, the listener. She visits for a month at a time, offering encouragement and emotional support.

Sometimes this support springs up naturally and spontaneously. In other situations, it's good to have a family planning conference early in the disease process. This will help identify and coordinate the skills family members can contribute as the disease progresses and their loved one's needs increase.

• Contributing to loved ones' financial needs is one way some relatives can share in the caring burden. Caring is expensive. Even if most of the expense is covered by the National Health or Social Services there are always items of extra expense; for example, some incontinence products, special foods, wheelchair repair, not to mention respite care.

• Family members living in other parts of the country often attend support groups themselves. This gives them a more realistic picture of what the primary carer is coping with and what their loved one is suffering. In addition, they can learn more about Alzheimer's disease by attending conferences and exchanging tapes, CDs or DVDs. Information they acquire can be shared across the miles.

• Never underestimate the value of letters and phone calls. For the primary carer the feeling of aloneness doesn't lessen as the years go by – no matter how involved one may be in the community or in a support group. Tangible notes of support and encouragement help maintain and strengthen family ties.

Caring really is a family affair. It is a time for sharing, caring and bearing each other's burdens in practical, tangible ways.

Little Ones

◄◄ *My five-year-old grandson loves his grandmother. When my daughter takes him to the nursing home to visit, he'll climb up on my wife's lap and kiss her. Then she'll smile, just like old times. He's the only one who can make her smile like that. He can be out in the hall and my wife will recognize his voice. She'll even yell at the nurses, 'That's my boy. Let him come!' My wife always calms down when he comes.*

I told my grandson that I wished we could have his grandmother back home again with us. You know what he said to me? He said, 'That's all right, Grandpa. Grandma's poorly. But that doesn't stop me from loving her.'

Newborns. Infants. Toddlers. School-age children. Teens. If you have any children in your family or can borrow some from your friends, they can be a source of joy for both you and your loved one. Relating to your loved one can likewise be a joy for them.

Occasionally, children will be frightened by their grandmother's or grandfather's bizarre behaviour, but most of the time they'll take it in their stride and accept it.

◄◄ *Mum and her four-year-old grandson get along just fine. To a four-year-old, everything is new in the world and everything is as it should be. Therefore, if Grandma is confused and forgetful, that's okay. It must be normal. We'll accept that behaviour. And so he does.*

When I hired home carers for my mother, one of the workers had two children, aged seven and nine. She brought them to work in the summer, and they always came over after school during the school year. Mum called them 'cute little fellers' (a phrase she also used when referring to the squirrels on our patio and even some of my older friends). But they didn't seem to mind. She also patted them on the head a lot and gave them hugs. They accepted her terms of endearment and responded in kind. To them, she was 'Gramma'.

Once I got home from work and discovered Mum and the two children hard at work on a special project that the children themselves had instituted. They'd brought over their colouring books and had also brought one for my mother. The three of them were having a great time colouring at the kitchen table. My mother the artist was once again at work.

As the months went by, Mum lost her ability to hold on to crayons. While her colouring lasted, it was a joy to watch her interact with the children for even short periods of time and to see the children care about her, accepting some of Mum's other behaviours as a normal part of life for an 'adopted grandmother' with Alzheimer's.

A week before my father died, one of the children wrote my mother a letter. It seems a fitting reminder of the importance of children in the lives of our loved ones – a reminder of what love is all about:

Dear Pearl
 Hi. How are you today. I love you a lot. You are my best Friend. You are more Than a Friend. You are Like a Grama to me and will all way be a Grama to me. Because I Love you so much you will allways Be in my Heart. You are so Loveable & soft and so warm and you allways will be in my Heart and in my Dreams. an so Does God Love you Like I Do. He Love's you to. He Does me and He Will allway's Look over you if I can't. He will allways watch over you pearl because I love you. and I love God to.
 From Tanya L. Rood to pearl

Chapter Eleven

Carer Support Systems

⏮ *Dad was very aggressive. He mellowed somewhat as he got older, but his temper got worse as the Alzheimer's disease came on. It was very hard on my mother. She was the type of person who would take everything and wouldn't fight back. But there were times when she would go into her room, shut the door, cry, and scream and scream – just to get rid of the tension. I don't know why she didn't have a nervous breakdown. Ten years, and no respite.*

As Alzheimer's disease progresses, most carers will need some short-term relief as well as more extended periods of respite. A volunteer or sitter might come in for several hours during the week initially. Friends or family members may also be willing to fill in for a day or a long weekend. An extended getaway, however, generally requires more formal arrangements. A number of options are available to carers depending on where you live, your financial situation and your needs.

Using all the available community services and care providers can make it possible for us to keep our loved one at home for as long as it is safe and desirable. They are not designed to totally take away our caring responsibilities, but to give us the short-term help we need to rest, regroup and recoup our personal strength and resources. We are then better equipped to manage at home when we return. Carers of relatives with dementia now have the right to request flexible working hours due to the Work and Families Act of 2006, which adjusts employment responsibilities around caring responsibilities in cooperation with employers.[1]

Home Care

Formal in-home services delivered through city, regional and community agencies include various types of support provided through voluntary agencies, Social Services and the National Health Service. Levels of care might include 'sitters', home helps/housekeepers, and more skilled nursing services as needs become more acute in the home and dementia is more advanced. Mealtime help may be provided through Meals-on-Wheels or other nutrition programmes that provide meals to people with disabilities.

Carers frequently cite the value of regularly scheduled home-care workers:

◄◄ *Helpers from a local home-care agency came in twice a week to give my husband a bath, shave him and give him his breakfast. After breakfast, they'd take him for a walk. It was so good to have a couple of hours to myself.*

◄◄ *I'm semi-retired and have a part-time teaching job two afternoons a week. I asked some volunteers from the Crossroads Care to come in when I finally realized I had to have someone with her when I was at work. My major support came from these volunteers.*

◄◄ *Home care was wonderful. It was my salvation. The girl who came was great. And I worked outside the home every day.*

My work was really my respite. I couldn't have stood being home all day long.

If you're looking for in-home services, the following tips may apply:

• Talk with other carers who have hired helpers. What services have they used? Were the services reliable and dependable?

• Ask about service information at your local GP or health centre. Ring Social Services, who can tell you what is available in your area and what type of help and financial assistance you and your loved one might be eligible for. Before you can access any statutory service you will be asked to consent to a care assessment. Community care assessments can be done by social workers on both carers and the cared-for person to determine needs and eligibility for various council-provided services at varying stages of dementia. It is also well worth contacting your local Alzheimer's group, Citizens Advice Bureau, Age Concern representative, Women's Royal Voluntary Service or other community organization and explaining your needs. Even if the people that you contact are unable to provide services directly, they should be able to refer you to agencies that can. Most people in the UK begin by receiving services through voluntary agencies and/or Social Services as long as both the carer and the person with Alzheimer's remain well and free from other health complications.

• Statutory health care can vary according to area, but may include a community psychiatric nurse (CPN), who can offer invaluable help and advice. A district nurse should be able to assist carers with coordinating bathing, dressing and other practical concerns in the home; basic help with the activities of daily living is generally given by trained care attendants hired by an agency that is supervised and monitored by Social Services. District nurses can provide direct nursing care that could include things like dressing changes or certain types of medication administration. Community night and twilight nursing services may be available to help with putting a confused elderly person to bed and providing care; this is generally available to people with advanced dementia and is on a time-limited basis.

• If you need home-care help following the hospital discharge of your loved one, contact the hospital's social worker as soon as possible. Usually you can do this through the nursing staff on the ward where your loved one is. Hospital staff can help you make post-hospital arrangements. Generally you will be asked to take part in meetings to discuss discharge plans. Be sure to agree upon the date and time of discharge and make sure you are satisfied with the plans for care and any additional help needed at home prior to the actual discharge. It is far easier to have anticipated services in place before you go home than to go home and then realize you need more help.

• Social Services will generally coordinate home-care services for you in the UK but there may be other options, such as hiring through an established, reputable agency. Agency services may include training and supervision of home-care workers, development of a specific plan of care, provision of substitute workers if the scheduled worker is ill, and provision of various levels of service ranging from cooking, cleaning and shopping to direct personal caring. Crossroads is an example of a voluntary agency that provides an attendant care service for families throughout England and Wales, providing millions of care hours to over 35,000 carers. It is designed to supplement the existing provision for care by Social Services. Enquire whether a Crossroads scheme operates in your area.

Turn the above advantages into questions for the agency when you ask about information and services. Written information should also be available about each agency's services, certification, fees and funding sources, and most services have websites with information carers need.

• Most people with dementia aged sixty-five and over are eligible for Attendance Allowance, and some for Mobility Allowance and Invalid Care Allowance. Attendance Allowance is not a means-tested benefit but is determined solely by care needs. Persons under age sixty-five with mild dementia in need of care supervision may claim Disability Living Allowance (DLA). Details of these benefits can be found in the *Disability Rights Handbook* (obtainable from the Disability Alliance and from the Alzheimer's Society; it is also available for order on-line). Benefits may change, and a Welfare Rights Adviser, who can be contacted through the local Citizens Advice Bureau, will be able to help you in these matters. The Alzheimer's Society has also established a Caring Fund from which small grants are made to those in need, as a supplement to state benefits.

Many home-care expenses are tax deductible for spouses and children who are primary carers. Be sure to save all medically related receipts and keep accurate records of expenses.

• You may also hire on an individual basis. Many men and women with kind hearts and good personal care skills are looking for home-care jobs. Newspapers may contain adverts from home-care workers seeking independent employment. These workers may or may not be trained and have previous experience in home-care, nursing home or hospital settings, though training itself is not necessarily an indication of how reliable or how honest an informal carer will be. Avoid hiring over the phone. It's best to have applicants come to your home for a personal interview. Are they able to physically manage your loved one? Find out about any health problems. Will they need to do heavy lifting? Can they? Discuss fees (they will usually set an hourly rate) based on what they want, what you can afford and what you believe is the going rate in your area.

To minimize risks, ask prospective employees for several references, preferably from previous employers. Call them. A good employee will not mind this or feel that it's an intrusion. Communicate with other carers who may have hired help in the past. A 'carer grapevine' can let you know who's reliable and who's not.

• College and hospital nursing programmes may be a useful source of home-care help. Students are often looking for part-time employment. Sometimes they are also looking for a place to live, perhaps while they take a break from their studies. For two years I had a student live with us. In exchange for room and board and a negotiated salary she cared for my mother and enabled me to hold down a full-time job. She had weekends and evenings off but was always willing to help me out when I needed some extra time for myself.

Age Concern has published a fact sheet called *Finding Help at Home*, which is worth obtaining.[2] Another useful free fact sheet, *Help at Home*, and dozens of other helpful fact sheets on available services and costs for carers may be obtained from Counsel and Care, a national charity for older people, their families and their carers (see Appendix D). Call specific agencies for order information or see their website for on-line orders and many free downloadable files.

Adult Day Centres

'If only there had been a place where I could have left my mother for the day. I simply needed a day off now and then,' said one carer. There are such places. Adult day-care programmes provide socialization, a nutritious meal, and a structured and supervised environment with a wide range of activities.

Availability, criteria for eligibility and the cost of day-care services vary widely from area to area, but they are usually one of the most economical forms of help for the carer.

Most adult day centres are run by local authorities or voluntary groups; others may be affiliated with and located in geriatric hospitals or nursing homes. Some centres care for all older people with physical and intellectual impairment. Others are only for those with physical disabilities or people with dementia. Payment may be means-tested.

One job I held several years ago necessitated a two-hour drive once a month for management meetings. The meeting was in a fairly large city. I enquired about day-care options and found a centre, which catered exclusively to Alzheimer's sufferers, only a mile from our meeting place. So Mum went with me on the monthly trips. She loved the run and seemed to thrive in the centre's environment.

I loved it too: eight hours later I was only a few pounds poorer. Home care would have cost me four to five times as much for the twelve hours away from home.

If you do any travelling, think about this option and ring in advance to learn about available services.

Sheltered Housing

Sheltered housing is becoming increasingly popular in the UK. It is designed for people generally over the age of sixty and consists of a group of flats, houses or bungalows that can be rented or sometimes purchased. Properties are self-contained housing units with their own bathrooms and fitted kitchens. There is a twenty-four-hour emergency call centre assistance for security and each scheme has its own manager. There are over 25,000 sheltered housing schemes in the UK. Sheltered housing is available for both individuals and couples. Health-care and support services can be utilized in the same way as in one's own home; added benefits for carers can be the proximity of neighbours and various social activities available in this type of housing. Services and age requirements vary. ERoSH, the national housing consortium for sheltered and retirement housing, has a very helpful website carrying information about this option.[3]

Residential and Nursing Homes

Residential and nursing homes are another alternative. These are run by local authorities or voluntary groups or, increasingly, they are privately run. They provide live-in, twenty-four-hour help for the frail elderly and the elderly with health-care needs. A few exclusively take in people with Alzheimer's. Some may have a designated number of beds for people with dementia and offer varying levels of care. These settings can become an available long-term option for persons with advanced dementia when carers are no longer able to keep their loved one at home. Some homes may be willing to care for people during the day, on an occasional overnight, or for several weeks or a month of respite for needy carers. Your social service department will have an official listing, though you may need more information than this offers. Website information is available on many homes.[4] Once again, ask around.

Another option I discovered was the 'sitter/companion'. Many child minders don't mind another mouth to feed at lunchtime and, if an Alzheimer's sufferer is manageable and doesn't wander, would see him or her as a welcome addition to their home. This also provides an opportunity for children to interact with older people, an increasingly rare phenomenon for some families; children can also provide good company for the Alzheimer's sufferer.

I used this service once a week. I dropped Mum off in the morning, went to work at the nursing home and returned later in the evening, taking some time for myself. My refrigerator was covered with 'pictures for Pearl' that one little girl kept giving us. Ask around. Check references if you need to.

Extended Care Facilities

Extended care facilities are also being built that have a range of adaptive housing options for people with various health-care needs. A person with Alzheimer's would receive various support services and monitoring. These arrangements are very popular in the US where they are often run by churches or voluntary agencies. People can move from one level of care to another as needs change; for example, from independent to assisted living to skilled care.

Other Alternatives

You may also want to consider some of these alternative options for the care of your loved one:

• The Holiday Care Service is a registered charity providing free information and advice on holidays for people with special needs. Contact them direct for their booklet *Care for Carers* and a range of other useful information for carers. Their address is in Appendix D.

• An exchange programme with other carers in your support group may be possible. It may not be any more difficult or time consuming to care for two or even three people with Alzheimer's than to care for one. In fact, there may be less care involved.

At the various day centres and residential homes I've either used or visited, I've seen that people with Alzheimer's have a language all of their own; they often communicate very well with each other. In fact, they may find it a relief to care for each other and talk to each other, and the carer's burden is lessened.

• For people with severe advanced dementia, hospital day care that includes nursing care, needed therapies and lunch at a day hospital may be an option. This is a valuable service for carers who work or need some respite during the day. This option is specific to people with advanced dementia who have various health needs. Attendance might be limited to once or twice a week.[5]

Keep Searching

Some carers have tried a number of the foregoing options and have had negative experiences. This is to be expected. We know that caring for someone with Alzheimer's is not easy. Not everyone can do it.

We needn't let one or even two or three rough experiences sour us to all substitute carers. Sooner or later we'll end up with a good match and probably wonder how we ever managed without the support of that particular home-care agency, volunteer sitter or day-care programme.

That's as it should be as we shift the caring responsibility on to someone else's shoulders for a while and take a needed break.

Chapter Twelve

Our Tangled Emotions

⏮ *I remember sitting in the kitchen with my two-year-old,
feeling miserable, when a song about a woman who had died
started playing on the radio. I started sobbing.*

*My emotions were all bottled up inside. That song
triggered them. I went outside, sat on the steps for half an
hour and cried and cried. I couldn't stop. There was all this
pent-up emotion.*

I knew it was because of my mother.

Our emotional responses to Alzheimer's are often as mixed up and
tangled as the minds of our loved ones. Sometimes we need help to
sort through them and straighten them out.

Fear, anxiety, guilt, anger and depression are the primary
emotions carers experience. But the full picture needn't look so
bleak. What we may perceive as negative emotions are a natural, if
uncomfortable, response to the loss of our loved one. The one we
love may still be alive and present, but not as the person we once
knew. What we are doing, in fact, is *grieving*. And grief is healthy
and normal.

Granger Westberg, in his popular book *Good Grief*, wrote about
the emotions people feel when facing the loss of a loved one. He
noted that there are good and bad ways to grieve, healthy and
unhealthy emotions to experience. Grief is a 'road the majority of
humans must travel in order to get back into the mainstream of life'.[1]
That applies to carers.

To be free from worry and anxiety in the face of uncertainty,
to be at peace with our loved ones without feeling resentful or
resigned – these are healthy signs that we have come to terms with

our conflicting emotions. They show that we are truly experiencing 'good' grief.

Fears and Anxieties

Fear and anxiety are common emotional reactions when a loved one is diagnosed with Alzheimer's. They are strongest among children of parents with Alzheimer's.

The question 'Is Alzheimer's disease hereditary?' is asked by every son and daughter. We pray the answer is no. We fear the answer is yes. Fear and anxiety may increase if we know our family history.

> ◄◄ *I think it may be the fourth generation for my mother. Her mother died when my mother was sixteen. We're sure it was Alzheimer's. My mother's grandmother had the same symptoms. Judging from the family anecdotes we've been gathering, a great-uncle had symptoms too.*

The fear becomes even greater if we, too, become forgetful.

> ◄◄ *Sometimes I forget the names of people I should know, and that terrifies me. My wife sees the look that comes over my face and she says, 'Now, don't start getting upset.'*

Many carers cope by joking about the possibility of Alzheimer's. Others use their knowledge to plan for the future.

> ◄◄ *My two sisters and I crack jokes about how we'll be the old Alzheimer's gals. We'll get a home together.*

> ◄◄ *I'm not really afraid of getting Alzheimer's. If I do, I hope I have enough lucid moments in the beginning so that I'll have time to make plans and take care of everything. I certainly don't sit around and worry. I do, occasionally, think about planning for the future.*

> ◄◄ *I kid about it with my housemate sometimes. She'll say to me, 'You're acting funny again. Sign the paper.' We make a joke of it.*

I did tell her that, if I ever start acting as my father did, I want to sign the paper so someone will have power of attorney over me.

Sometimes the more we know about the disease, the less we're able to cope with it. Other people can help put our fears and anxieties in perspective.

⏮ *I read some information about Alzheimer's disease that said I had a good chance of getting Alzheimer's because my mother had it. Then I went to a conference where they talked about the heredity factor. I was so depressed when I came home, I spent the next four days in bed.*

A friend said, 'Are you going to make your husband and your children miserable for the next twenty years just because you think you might get it? You'll ruin your lives. And besides, you could get hit by a bus tomorrow. A plane could fall from the sky. You simply can't worry about getting this disease.'

Are fear and anxiety justified? Is Alzheimer's hereditary? What are the risks to children whose parents have Alzheimer's and to future generations?

Studies have demonstrated an increased risk of developing Alzheimer's among those who have Alzheimer's in their family. Those closest to the person with Alzheimer's are at a slightly higher risk than relatives several generations removed. According to one study, the overall risk of acquiring Alzheimer's disease is about four times greater if you have a first-degree relative (parents, siblings, children) with dementia. Although this risk to even first-degree relatives is still very small, it increases as people reach their seventies and eighties. Some relatives of people with Alzheimer's do develop dementias in later life. Others do not. In a few families Alzheimer's appears to be inherited more frequently than normal; researchers have identified genetic mutations in these families and are exploring this as a further avenue for research.[2]

Researchers are also looking for links between Alzheimer's and similar diseases. One area of genetic exploration is related to Down's syndrome (also known as Down syndrome), a hereditary condition accompanied by an extra partial or complete chromosome 21 that causes profound mental impairment. Down's syndrome is named after British physician John Langdon Down, who first described it in 1866; in 1959 French physician Jerome Lejeune identified the actual chromosomal anomaly.

The possible genetic thread linking Alzheimer's disease and Down's syndrome is the presence of a large number of senile plaques and neurofibrillary tangles present in the brain tissue of both people with Alzheimer's and people with Down's syndrome.

Autopsies on people over the age of forty with Down's syndrome showed evidence of the characteristic plaques and tangles of Alzheimer's disease – even if they didn't show signs of Alzheimer's when they were alive. This finding has sparked considerable interest and activity in genetic research that may one day help to uncover a cause and more effective treatments for Alzheimer's. People with Down's syndrome who develop dementia may require the same type of support as anyone else with Alzheimer's and exhibit similar symptoms. Many parents of children with Down's are also older themselves as prevalence at birth increases with maternal age; they will benefit from information on both Down's and Alzheimer's care and support services.[3]

It is possible to be referred to a genetic counsellor through your GP if you are concerned about the inherited form of Alzheimer's disease in your family. Rather than fear the genetic implications, however, we should welcome scientific advances and encourage the research that may help subsequent generations. (See Appendix C for more detailed information on genetic research and Alzheimer's.)

Hope for future generations may seem scant comfort when you are personally struggling with the reality of Alzheimer's disease. But if God provides rain for the earth and food for the animals, he can and will provide for us. He can give us the strength to be carers today and to face the future with peace.

The Guilt Trip

Psychiatrist Karl Menninger, in his book W*hatever Became of Sin?*, described a man who stood on a busy street corner and repeated one word aloud, over and over again. The word was *guilty*. Each time the man said 'Guilty,' he'd point at a passerby. The accused people hesitated, looked away, then glanced furtively at each other – as if they actually felt guilty.[4]

Carers may feel a lot like those poor pedestrians. Whatever we say, wherever we go, whatever we do, we can't escape the pointing finger. If we don't think others are pointing it at us, we point it at ourselves. It's a no-win situation.

What makes us feel guilty? Dozens of things.

We feel guilty about our attitude towards our loved one's confusion, agitation and behaviour.

⏮ *I felt guilty every minute of the day. Not so much for the way I treated my mother, but for the things I thought about her.*

I didn't shout or scream, but I certainly felt like it at times. Her agitation, and especially the repetitiveness, drove me nuts.

I usually coped by walking out of the room, leaving my mother in her chair to talk to herself. I suppose you might call that neglect, but it was the only way I could handle my emotions.

⏮ *I was never outright nasty to my wife. I didn't physically abuse her. But I acted as if she didn't exist. She'd ask me a question for the twenty-fifth time in one morning and I'd just walk away.*

Ignoring her became a habit.

I felt guilty about it, a nagging, clawing kind of guilt.

Our behaviour can bother us when we finally vent our pent-up emotions and verbally or even physically lash out at our loved ones in a carer's version of a catastrophic reaction.

◄◄ *I would be so very mean to my husband. I'd say cutting, hurtful things to him. I couldn't seem to stop myself. I was so frustrated.*

◄◄ *I would get angry with my wife and feel bad later. I don't think you can help that. You're driven to extremes, then afterwards you're sorry.*

Once my wife bit me so hard I turned around and bit her on the shoulder. She had so many clothes on it didn't hurt her at all. It was just a sudden reaction on my part. Then I felt guilty.

The decision to place a loved one in a nursing home is often fraught with guilt, compounded by the promises we may have made to 'never, ever do such a thing'.

◄◄ *I think the hardest thing for me was taking my husband to the nursing home. He was still lucid enough to realize we were taking him away from his home, and he said, 'I worked so hard all my life. Why are you doing this to me?' You can imagine how I felt, how I still feel.*

◄◄ *Father used to say, 'Don't ever put me in a nursing home. Take me out in the field and shoot me before you put me in one of those places.'*

So we told him we'd never do it. And then, one day, we did it.

◄◄ *I've read that people have taken care of their loved ones at home for seventeen years.*

So I felt guilty for not keeping him at home.

I still feel guilty whenever I visit him, especially if he's alert.

But what could I do? I'm eighty-nine years old.

Wishing a parent, spouse, sister or brother dead and out of their misery is not an uncommon source of guilt.

◄◄ *When my brother was still driving, I thought that maybe he'd drive off the cliff at the back of our house and it would be over for him. It would end his suffering. I never told anyone I had those thoughts.*

◄◄ *Once my father was lost and my brother found him wandering down by the river. When he came home, my brother said to me, 'I had the most horrible thoughts when we were searching. I hoped that Dad might have fallen in the river and that it was all over for him. I felt so guilty for thinking that way.'*

Neglected responsibilities make us feel guilty – the floors to mop, the lawn to mow, letters to answer and the bills to pay.

◄◄ *I know my house is a wreck and I've let things pile up. Sometimes I get overwhelmed by depression. Most of the time I just feel guilty because I think I should be able to get my act together and keep things in order: my father, my house, my life.*

◄◄ *Our neighbours must think they live next to an abandoned building. The grass is two feet high. Garden work is always at the bottom of my priority list, and I feel ashamed of the way my house looks. Inside as well as outside.*

Unmet family obligations and needs can create guilt for us.

◄◄ *My husband was a brick through it all. Sometimes I wonder why he didn't ask for a divorce. I certainly didn't meet many of his needs for a whole year after my mother moved in with us. Any of his needs, if you know what I mean.*

◄◄ *It was hard on the children to grow up in the same house with a grandparent who had Alzheimer's. They never complained, but I know it was hard.*
We couldn't do anything together as a family, because someone had to stay at home and watch Dad. I don't think I

have any pictures from a family vacation. Holidays never happened. I feel bad about that.

Psychologists may tell us this carer guilt is false, related to the unrealistic expectations we have of ourselves. This may be true. But simply *calling* it false guilt doesn't help, and sorting out false guilt from true guilt when we're overwhelmed by caring responsibilities can seem impossible.

◄◄ *At home we tried every day to give Dad a bath or just wash him, but he'd always fight. When we took Dad to the nursing home, he had dirt in the creases of his neck. I was embarrassed.*

When I visited him and looked at his neck, it was clean. I said, 'Thank God,' but I was embarrassed again!

Sometimes we need other people to help us sort through our feelings and emotions. A friend, members of a carer support group, counsellors and clergy can all be valuable sounding boards.

Yet when we're all talked out, supported, analyzed and back home again, we may find that things haven't really changed. Our guilt hasn't walked away. We still respond the same way to the same situations. Guilt can continue to incapacitate us emotionally and physically. It threatens to eat up our energy, buffet our bodies, and force us into self-condemnation and depression.

Guilt, even false guilt, is never benign. And, unfortunately, false guilt can be a smoke screen. It can effectively hide an underlying problem we have apart from our caring experiences. That problem is *true* guilt.

Good News

None of us is perfect in all our actions and attitudes. If we deal with any type of guilt superficially by denying it or rationalizing it, we can continue to struggle alone. But I believe if we admit to God our deep-down failings and regrets we can experience genuine forgiveness.

The freedom that comes from being forgiven is more than simply not feeling guilty. It is the experience of new life and the promise of life to come. It is the realization that it's possible to have joy in the midst of mourning, hope in the midst of despair. It is knowing that the experience of caring does not have to devastate us. That is indeed good news.

Chapter Thirteen

Hot But Not Burned Up

Just prior to becoming a carer for my own parents I was working in a nursing home in Illinois as both a spiritual-care coordinator and a nurse in charge of a unit. I loved my job, I loved the area, and I was in love. The fact that he wasn't equally in love with me was something I thought would work itself out in time. I was really looking forward to my future.

Then came the phone call.

'Sharon,' said my aunt, my father's youngest sister, 'you know you've always said to let you know if there were any problems on the home front. Well, there are. With your mother. I think it's time you moved back home.' That was not news I wanted to hear.

I knew for years that my mother was having 'a bit of a memory problem'. I attributed it to her recent retirement, failing eyesight and my dad's sudden onset of adult diabetes, an event that seemed to throw my mother into a state of confusion and anxiety. Alzheimer's disease was the furthest thing from my mind. I wasn't even sure I could spell it and it was not yet a common diagnosis in many nursing homes in the US.[1] I received a lot of advice from friends and colleagues. Even the administrator of the nursing home called me into her office. She gave me a very comforting lecture on how I needed to think about my needs, my future, my job. 'Perhaps you should call your father and talk to him about the possibility of nursing-home placement,' she suggested. Take a short leave of absence, get things sorted out at home, then come back. Neat. Simple. Just what I wanted to hear.

That was not, however, what I was supposed to do. God, it seemed, had other plans for my life. He made them clear in no uncertain terms one night when I was reading the Bible.

In a passage from the book of Mark, Jesus was speaking to the religious leaders of the day. He was talking to them about their responsibility to their parents, and he called them hypocrites. They apparently gave money for temple offerings while their parents went hungry. They were, Jesus said, worshipping God in vain.

I felt convicted and doomed. I packed my bags – not eagerly, not happily – and drove home.

For the next few years I helped my father care for my mother. I either lived at home or shuffled back and forth between my parents' home and an apartment in a nearby city where I found a nursing job. Life seemed an unending merry-go-round of work, work and more work as Mum's symptoms got worse, my father developed cancer, and I had to face the fact that I was probably back home for good, constantly caring and still very much single.

I was also very angry with God.

My own primary support system had always been my church. I stopped going. The Bible had always been my point of strength. I stopped reading it. Prayer had always been my source of encouragement. I stopped praying.

For months I continued being angry, isolated and miserable. Then I finally came to terms with my feelings and began dealing with them constructively.

God isn't always the target of our anger. Sometimes we're angry at Alzheimer's itself, a disease we barely understand and certainly can't control.

◄◄ *I was angry at this disease that was destroying my father's mind. I was angry because life wasn't turning out the way I'd envisioned for my parents.*

◄◄ *I quit smoking so I wouldn't get lung cancer. I changed my diet so I wouldn't have a heart attack. And here comes this disease that I have absolutely no control over, I can't do anything to prevent it. I realize no matter how healthy my lifestyle is, I won't be able to stop it or do anything about it if I get it. And because my mother has it, I look at myself as being a sitting duck.*

> *It angers me. I know anger isn't going to do me any*
> *good, but it makes me so cross.*

Sometimes our anger is directed at our loved ones, then at ourselves because we don't feel good about our angry outbursts. We want to change, but we struggle.

> ◄◄ *We were angry with my mother for the things she said*
> *and did. It would be so frustrating. She would ask the same*
> *questions over and over again until my father thought he'd go*
> *out of his mind. What day is it? What day is it? What month is*
> *it? What month is it? The same questions over and over.*
>
> *Dad would say, 'For Pete's sake, I told you the answer to*
> *that ten times already.' Then he'd go into the bedroom and*
> *slam the door.*

> ◄◄ *There's always a tendency, especially if there are other*
> *people around, to let your best side show, though inside you*
> *know things are different. I didn't want my patience to be a*
> *mask I was putting on.*
>
> *When I got those feelings of anger and impatience, I*
> *didn't like it. Daddy knew he was irritating me. He'd try*
> *to apologize for something that wasn't his fault. I got very*
> *upset with myself for being angry and impatient with him*
> *when he'd ask me the same thing for the hundredth time.*
>
> *When I got that way, I'd go into the bedroom and talk to*
> *God. I'd say, 'Help me to be patient. Help me to remember.*
> *Help me to show Daddy the patience I'd want someone to*
> *show me.'*

Primary carers may feel they are the only ones who really care about their loved ones. Anger at other members of the family, who 'never call, never visit, never show any concern', is common.

> ◄◄ *I don't understand why my wife's brother never visits. For*
> *ten years she's had Alzheimer's. For five years she's been in the*
> *nursing home. He's never visited her there once. Not once.*

·   *Part Three:* Caring for Yourself

In hospitals and nursing homes, anger is sometimes directed at doctors, nurses or other health-care staff.

> ◄◄ *I got furious at some of the things the health-care assistants would say or do. You can't treat people like cattle, but that's the way they behaved at times. Especially at mealtimes. I'd see a few of them shovelling the food into patients' mouths and hear them say things like, 'If you don't eat this they're going to send you to the hospital and put a tube down your nose.'*

Sometimes we even vent our frustrations on the furniture:

> ◄◄ *I never told my husband this, but the reason the mirror is broken in the bathroom is because I slammed the bathroom door so hard the mirror broke. I told him I was trying to kill a wasp with a broom handle. I think he believed me. I was just so ashamed of myself for getting so angry that I'd actually started destroying the furniture.*

Not all expressions of anger are healthy. Our angry outbursts can hurt other people. They can also make us feel guilty and ashamed of ourselves. But the emotion of anger itself is not always unhealthy or destructive. Anger can be a legitimate response to justifiable causes.

What makes us angry? And why? These are the two key questions.

Anger at God

'Whenever there is suffering, whether physical pain or mental anguish, man-at-his-best will do his best to help. But his powers are so limited. God's power, so they say, is unlimited. So why doesn't He do something?' wrote Hugh Silvester in *Arguing with God*.[2]

British author C. S. Lewis, in *A Grief Observed*, also asked 'Why?' when his wife was diagnosed with a fatal illness:

> ◄◄ *What chokes every prayer and every hope is the memory of all the prayers (she) and I offered and all the false hopes*

we had. Not hopes raised merely by our own wishful thinking;
hopes encouraged, even forced upon us, by false diagnoses, by
x-ray photographs, by strange remissions, by one temporary
recovery that might have ranked as a miracle. Step by step we
were 'led up the garden path'.[3]

A bit earlier (three to four thousand years earlier), a man named Job
had also asked the *why* question as he sat on an ash heap, stricken
by boils, grieving about his own physical suffering and the deaths of
his ten children. The writer of the book of Job says Job bitterly cried
out against the apparent injustice of God in light of his own physical
and emotional suffering:

I am tired of living. Listen to my bitter complaint. Don't
condemn me, God. Tell me! What is the charge against me?
  Is it right for you to be so cruel? To despise what you
yourself have made? And then to smile on the schemes of
wicked men?

Today, many people with Alzheimer's, and their carers, are still
asking, 'Why?'

⏮ *My wife can't understand why everything happened to*
her the way it did. She said that if you believe in God, then
things should be nice in life, even in old age. But things didn't
turn out nice. They turned out terrible.

⏮ *When my mother got Alzheimer's, I told God and the*
church goodbye. I reckoned if there was a God he could have
prevented it. And if God didn't allow it to happen, maybe he
caused it to happen. So who needed him?
  It's so easy to blame God, especially if he's responsible
for everything. I have a convenient place to put my anger:
God's to blame. God's at fault. It has taken me years to get
over my anger.

Why *doesn't* God do something about Alzheimer's disease? Why does
he allow it to happen in the first place? Isn't he supposed to be good?

There's one school of thought that says you shouldn't argue about the nature of God when a person is sick or dying. But when we are seriously or terminally ill or when someone we love is suffering or dying, that's the time we struggle most with these kinds of questions. In reality, it's a time when many of our other beliefs are tried and tested, formed and reformed as well, questions about God's goodness, power and even his very existence. My own struggles with the goodness of God revolved as much around my own frustrated plans and desires as they did around my mother's disease and the devastating effects it had on both her and my father. For me, it wasn't so much an issue of the goodness of God in general as it was the goodness of God in particular. When things are going well for me (by my standards) I may rarely question God's goodness. God's goodness can become an issue, however, when I'm faced with a personal crisis. Why, God, don't you do something for *my* loved one? Why don't you do something for *me*?

Turning our thoughts away from ourselves can help us put our own situation in perspective. It can help us realize we are not alone in our grief. Others walk that road too, others who have concluded that even though they don't know all the answers, God has not abandoned them, as the following carer noted:

⏮ *I was angry at God for several years after my mother was diagnosed with Alzheimer's disease. Then I started going back to church. I decided to go for the sake of the kids, not so much because I'd got over my anger.*

On the first day back, I saw a woman whose son had been killed in a plane crash and a woman in her thirties whose husband had died of a heart attack. I realized that though they'd been through all that suffering, they still believed in God. I started crying. I cried through the whole service. That's what brought me back to God.

It is okay to be angry. It is not okay to stay angry for ever. Christopher Allison, in *Guilt, Anger and God*, wrote about the need to move beyond anger:

◄◄ *It is strange that the cultural taboo against admitting anger toward God has... made us regard it as shocking and something to be suppressed. The thought of expressing our anger toward God in worship is scandalous to many. Yet this is an indication of how far we have departed from scriptural guides. The Psalms... are generously sprinkled with anger toward God for injustice on earth. Anger certainly is a major theme in the book of Job... Our sickness is our destructive anger. Our medicine is God's taking our anger. If we do not give it to him we are not healed of it.*[4]

Pain and suffering are not part of God's original plan. Disease and death were not part of the good world he created. Alzheimer's is *not* normal.

Yet those with Alzheimer's and those who care for them can have hope – not that we'll necessarily be delivered from this present suffering, but that we have someone to walk through it with us. No matter how hotly our anger may burn.

Anger at Others

As Alzheimer's takes its toll on our emotions, we will be tempted to lash out at those around us, venting our anger at the expense of other people. To keep our cool, we may need to think about safety valves.

A safety valve releases excess pressure. Pressure cookers have them. When pressure inside becomes more than the pan can bear, an automatic valve on top releases the steam.

Carers need safety valves too. We need to know how to release our anger and frustration in *constructive* ways. We may also need to plan for the future and take preventive measures at the start to keep the pressure from building to explosive levels. Excessive pressure build-up for the carer can result in explosions of uncontrolled anger.

Emergency measures for immediate situations may include some of the following:

• When tempted to verbally or even physically lash out at your loved one, pull yourself together and count to ten. If necessary, walk away from the situation. If you need to vent your anger, pound a pillow, clean out a cupboard, scrub a floor, chop wood. Avoid throwing and kicking things. Caring is expensive enough without having to replace the furniture.

• Put yourself in your loved one's situation. Ask yourself, 'How would I like to be treated?'

The following paragraphs offer practical suggestions for defusing anger in less volatile situations.

Distraction is a useful tool we can use with our loved ones and ourselves. Distraction is anything that gives mental amusement, relaxation or diversion.

Laughing at a situation instead of getting angry or frustrated can be one way of lessening pressure and a means of distraction. You're laughing not at your relative, but at the situation. Laughter lets off steam. Your loved one may also appreciate a good laugh at times. I laughed with my mother a lot. I think it helped us both to remember that life was not meant to be gloom and doom; it's meant to be lived and enjoyed, even the difficult moments.

The apostle Paul had good advice for anxious and angry people: rejoice, be gentle, talk to God about your needs. All these things can bring peace of heart and peace of mind. In addition he encourages us to fill our minds with thoughts that are true, pure, lovely and praiseworthy. All of these thoughts make for peaceful meditation. Martin Luther described this kind of meditation another way. He talked about letting our 'thoughts go for a walk'.[5] The scene before you may be one of utter chaos, but *you* don't have to be an internal wreck. When tempted to explode, turn your mind to some happy memory from the past or think about an anticipated event. Meditate on a psalm, a hymn, a quotation or some other beautiful aspect of the natural created world. I took my mum for many walks, pushing her wheelchair on the dirt road near a lake where I had moved us to after my father's death. It was a time for both of us to drink in the beauty of nature and it had a calming effect on us both. I chose the location purposefully.

When tempted to lash out at other loved ones, such as relatives who never call or visit, think about the possible reasons for their actions. Are they, too, having difficulty dealing with their loved one's illness? Do they need you to reach out to them and 'give them permission' to share their own feelings of grief? Talking to your relatives about your feelings may be the best thing you can do for you all. And if talking's not possible, forgive. Carrying a load of resentment inside will only be destructive.

If nursing-home staff or other health professionals do things or say things that anger us, we should let them know about it. Not by exploding in rage, but by talking to them about their attitude, their behaviour and the things we believe are negative responses. Sometimes, because of our own guilt, we may overreact and get angry about things that are a normal part of nursing-home life. At other times, our anger may be justified. Others may need help in viewing the situation through your eyes, the eyes of a carer. We all need to be sensitive to each other and to work together as a team. Honest, open communication can help make this possible.

There are also a number of preventive measures we can take to make the build-up of anger less of a problem. Because these measures are also good cures for depression, they are covered in the following chapter.

Anger at Alzheimer's

It's normal to be angry at Alzheimer's. It's a thief, a murderer, a destroyer of minds.

While ranting and raving at it won't do anyone any good, there are positive things we can do to help us feel more in command of this seemingly uncontrollable disease. We can channel our anger in practical ways by getting involved in the fight against Alzheimer's and other related dementias.

You may feel, as a carer, that you have neither the time nor the emotional or physical energy needed for involvement on any other level than an occasional support group meeting. If you do have the energy, however, here are a few suggestions. Some can be done individually, others with a group:

• Help plan a seminar to educate other carers, health professionals and the general public about Alzheimer's. Your own support group could join with others in your region or plan with local hospitals, nursing colleges or community service agencies.

• Order a box of supplies from the Alzheimer's Society and set up a table or booth to distribute them at community health fairs and town fêtes. I was the public relations person for our local Alzheimer's support group. For several years I sat in a booth at our local county fair, distributed literature and answered questions. I knew there was a need for this when one woman who was walking by the booth stopped suddenly, turned to look at our sign and said to her husband, 'You know, George, I think that's the disease our neighbour's cow died of.' Some other good sources for literature are found in Appendix D.

• Develop and distribute a newsletter for your area if none is available.

• Offer yourself as a speaker to nursing homes, hospitals, college classes on ageing and health, civic groups and churches. This could be a formal presentation, a simple question-and-answer session, or a panel presentation.

• Ask a reporter from a local newspaper to write an article about Alzheimer's or submit one yourself. Raise public awareness of the disease and let people know what's available in the community.

• Support the Alzheimer's Society financially. Many carers also encourage giving to the society at the time of the death of a loved one as a lasting memorial.

• Get involved politically. Be informed about local and national legislation related to caring issues and funding for Alzheimer's research. Write letters to your Member of Parliament as well as to government ministers for health and social services. You can also let your views be known to your local councillor, the chairperson of the local health authority, the chairperson of the local Social Services and the Community Health Council for your area. Remember that the people who hold the purse strings at all levels of government need to hear from the people who know about the disease. The people most in the know are carers.

Major issues to speak up on include financial support for carers. State benefits are currently inadequate in terms of paying for institutional care and meeting carers' needs. Many people believe that they should be at least at the level of the state pension. You may wish to support Carers UK, an organization of carers that supports home caring in many ways and seeks to influence policy that directly affects carers and their loved ones. Another vital issue concerns the availability and standard of care services, especially respite care. It must be recognized that regular short breaks are needed for carers, at least one half day per week. Alzheimer's also needs to be more widely acknowledged as a terminal illness so that people with Alzheimer's can qualify for the terminal illness level of Income Support. This would benefit patients, carers, and hospitals and homes that are often underfunded.

Most worthy causes became causes because someone got angry. A loved one was killed by a drunk driver or abducted from a school playground, died of cancer or suffered from Alzheimer's disease. The war against Alzheimer's is far from over. We all need to get involved in some battles and channel our anger in constructive ways.

Chapter Fourteen

Down But Not Out

Elaine remembered when she loved her job. When it had been, in fact, her respite. But lately the tensions at work were unbearable. There was always the constant backbiting and bickering. And there were the stupid, hateful things the other women said about their husbands. If they only knew, Elaine thought bitterly. They should be grateful they have husbands.

They should come home with me, she thought. See what it's like to live with a husband who doesn't even know your name. They'd begin to appreciate what they've got in a hurry. I wonder if anyone would take me up on the offer if I did invite them home.

Home. Thinking of home, Elaine wondered how the new home-care helper was getting on. The previous one lasted only a week. She handed in her resignation to the agency the day Stephen locked her out of the house. He had unlocked the kitchen door in the morning and run out into the back garden. When the helper ran after him, Stephen ran back into the kitchen, slamming and locking the door.

The woman spent two hours pleading with Stephen to let her in. But Stephen just stood there, smiled and waved at her. When the helper saw him turn the gas on under an empty frying pan, she had the presence of mind to run to the neighbour's house and call the police. And then she rang her agency.

Despite the problems, Elaine didn't know what she'd have done without the home-care agency. The helpers had been so good to Stephen. One of them even joked about losing ten pounds the first week she cared for him. It made Elaine feel guilty, until the carer reassured her it was the best thing to happen to her figure in years.

But people in their fifties weren't supposed to *need* minders. They weren't supposed to get Alzheimer's disease. Cancer maybe, or diabetes, or a heart attack. Terrible things, too, but all potentially treatable. Not Alzheimer's. Not this horrible disease that turned you into some kind of hyperactive child.

When had it first begun? When did she first notice the signs?

It wasn't until Stephen received the letter from the school requesting his resignation that reality finally hit her.

The absent-minded professor, the kids called Stephen at school. At first it showed in little things. He would correct their essays but forget to give them marks. Then he went through one term without giving an exam at all. The students never told. The school governors accidentally found out about Stephen's memory lapses when one of the governors overheard his daughter talking to a friend about the strange and wonderful chemistry teacher.

Finally the day came when, in the middle of the chemistry lab, Stephen threw a beaker at a student in a fit of frustration. Fortunately, the only thing in the beaker was water. It was supposed to have been acid, but Stephen had forgotten the formula.

Now Elaine could look back and see other changes. There were initially problems with words. Stephen always seemed to be searching to find the noun or the phrase to end a sentence. It started to drive Elaine crazy. Half the time she didn't know what he was talking about.

And there were personality changes. The frustration. The angry outbursts for no apparent reason.

She remembered the Saturday morning when Stephen went to the shops for a pint of milk and returned six hours later. She had really laid into him, accusing him of everything under the sun. And Stephen just looked at her, then went into the bedroom, slammed and locked the door and stayed there until after dark. That happened just before they got the letter from the school governors.

Two years later, here they were. Alone in a world where nothing made sense any more.

Maybe she should have listened to her mother and had a child. But no. She and Stephen had both felt that all they wanted was each other and their careers. They were planning to take a trip around the world in three more years. No strings. No children. Each other.

Elaine opened her desk and reached for her bag. Time to go home. Home to the man she still loved beyond distraction but who didn't even know her name.

Facing Depression

Depression is an emotion we all experience as carers. It can range from sadness to profound sorrow, sometimes accompanied by physical symptoms. It is triggered by many things for the carer, and is associated with the profound changes we see in our loved ones and the many losses we experience over time related to our relationship with them.

Depression can descend like a weight when we realize that we are no longer known by our loved one:

⏮ *They say it gets easier but I don't believe it. Each time I go to see my wife it gets harder for me. It's as if I were a total stranger. I hug her and kiss her and talk to her, but she doesn't know me. She doesn't know what's going on.*

Depression can also be related to the death of expectations, like that experienced by Elaine in the scenario that introduced this chapter. Many who seem to have a bright and productive future suddenly see that future destroyed by a diagnosis:

⏮ *The real irony was that a week after my father was diagnosed, he got a letter from a company he used to work for asking him if he'd consider being the executive director.*

Depression can be related to the fact that our loved one is not able to experience the joys of grandparenting:

⏮ *If I started crying, my son would toddle upstairs, get some tissue, come and sit on my lap, and pat me as if to say everything would be okay. The fact that my mother had this beautiful little grandchild who was comforting me because of her made my depression worse. I wanted so much for them to know each other, but I knew it could never happen.*

Depression is often related to the anxiety, suffering and hopelessness our loved one is experiencing. Their confusion doesn't eliminate emotions like fear and frustration. They may also have a sense of meaninglessness, and suicidal thoughts that can be accompanied by actions.

◄◄ *I've had people say to me, especially nurses, 'Don't worry about your father. You're suffering more than he is.'*

I cannot believe that. I see my father's emotions. I see his facial expressions and his behaviour. I say to myself, no one can tell me he's not feeling something.

I don't believe that he's living in his own peaceful little world and that he doesn't know anything or anybody and he's not suffering. I see signs of anxiety and frustration. I see the look on his face when he wants to say something and can't get the words out.

I will never be convinced he's not suffering.

◄◄ *My wife used to have a tremendous will, not wanting to let anything get the better of her. Then, just before Christmas, she gave up.*

◄◄ *In the spring my husband tried to commit suicide. He got out one night when I was asleep. When I woke up, I called the police and we went searching. We finally found him up on the railway tracks. There was a train coming. He said to the police, 'Leave me alone. Leave me alone. I want to die. I have a right to kill myself if I want to.'*

Sometimes when we're depressed, the underlying problem is really our anger. One common definition of depression is 'anger turned inward'.

◄◄ *For months I was depressed. My wife finally said to me, 'Honey, I don't think your problem is depression. I think you're just angry at what happened to your father.' She was right.*

Role-reversals

My mother used to call me Sharon. Then it became 'Honey', the name she called me as a child. Pretty soon I became 'Mom' to her as her Alzheimer's progressed. And finally I became 'Gramma'.

For most people life is filled with roles. For carers, it's also filled with role-reversals. That can also contribute to depression.

◄◄ Just when I thought the nest was empty, I find it filled again. Not with grandchildren, but with my husband.

The role of a carer can be a blessing or a curse, depending on our attitude. It can cause us to wither away and die or it can help us to mature and grow emotionally and spiritually.

◄◄ I see the role change with both my parents as I handle their affairs. I handle everything for them. I'm their mouthpiece, their spokesperson.

As soon as I moved back home, my mother saw me as the one in charge.

But I never looked on my parents as children. I just believe that now, in their senior years, they need more help. And I can help them.

I prayed for years, when I was away from home, that God would give me an opportunity to care for my parents in their old age if they needed it. I've accepted it and am thankful for it.

Searching for the Light

In his chapter on depression and loneliness in the book *Good Grief*, Granger Westberg likens depression to a dreadfully dark day when the sun is blacked out by clouds. He says that people will always say, 'The sun isn't shining today.' But that's not true. The sun is shining, even when it appears not to be. Get on a plane, climb through the layer of clouds, and eventually you'll see that the sun *is* shining. And, says Westberg, someone will always make the remark, 'Too bad the people downstairs can't see this.'[1]

The sunshine. The light moments. We need to look for those light moments in our loved ones' lives and not be afraid to enjoy them.

◄◄ We have our jokes, our light moments. We laugh at some of the things Dad does. He's very funny sometimes. Like the day he set off the fire alarm in the nursing home. Or the day he decided to take a walk outside. He wheeled another resident

---

out of the door too. *The other man didn't want to go and was shouting 'No, no, no,' and carrying on. But Dad didn't care. It was a nice day for a trip.*

Dad always had this affectionate way of patting you on the behind. He did it to me not too long ago, and I said to Mum, 'There, he's his old self. He did it again.'

These little, light moments may last only a split second, but when they do appear they're good. They're very good.

Looking for the light moments is one way carers cope with depression. Preventive measures are another way to prevent the pressure from building up in our lives. They may not eliminate depression for us and our loved ones, but they can lighten the emotional load.

Maintaining Physical Fitness

If you spend half your day running around the neighbourhood in search of your relative or running up and down stairs ensuring their safety, you may be physically fit. Not all of us do this. Some loved ones are confined to wheelchairs and lead very sedentary lives. So do some carers.

The benefits of exercise in relation to stress reduction are well documented. When our large muscles are exercised, our involuntary muscles also relax. Stress is reduced. We have more energy. We feel better all over.

Here are some suggestions for maintaining your fitness.

• For me and for several other carers I interviewed, swimming is a key to tension reduction. It helps ease depression and is a good way of keeping aerobically fit.

When I became a full-time carer, I thought my year-round swimming days might be over. The nearby lake was perfect for summer swimming, but the winter months loomed dark and dreary. Then I spoke with the director of our local YMCA. 'Swim here,' he said. 'Your mother can come too.'

Mum's 'going to the pool' consisted of sitting downstairs in a deep and comfortable chair next to the TV and the front desk where there was always someone in attendance. The helpers agreed to keep an eye on her and would let me know if I was needed.

Mum was not agitated in this stage of the disease and was very content looking through old magazines until I returned. She also seemed to enjoy the children who ran around and sometimes stopped to talk to her. Any anger or depression I had when I went into the pool diminished or disappeared altogether after half an hour of laps.

Some carers hire in-home help if they aren't able to take their loved ones with them. Some have even learned to swim and have met new friends.

• If you're a runner or a walker, find a field or a track and take your loved one with you. Let him or her sit and watch you huff and puff. A wheelchair ride around the block a few times can also be good exercise for you and a good outing for your loved one. (Check with the Disabled Living Foundation Information Service, a surgical supply shop or on-line for types of chairs best suited for this. Many are very sturdy but portable as well. You will want a chair that is also light enough for you to lift in and out of your car. Sometimes this expense is at least partially reimbursable.)

• Golfing is another sport many couples have enjoyed in the dementia-free past. If so, don't think you have to give this up. Your loved one may enjoy riding in a golf cart or, like my mother, sitting in the clubhouse looking out of the window and waving to all the golfers. This only works if there are people around willing to keep a watchful eye out, as there were in the small rural club where I went. This carer-friendly golf club enabled me to relax and enjoy a round of golf for several summers when Mum was past the wandering stage and was content to sit in a chair.

Some people with Alzheimer's can continue to enjoy golf, tennis, bowling and other sports. They may no longer be able to keep score or play for as long as they used to, of course. But do continue to help them do the things they've always done for as long as they are able (if they can do them and not be frustrated by their diminished abilities).

• Maintain a balanced diet. This may seem obvious, but many carers (myself included) don't do it. A balanced diet includes food from the four basic food groups, the same as a balanced diet for those we care for (see chapter eight). In addition, the following recommendations should help us look better, feel better and be less fatigued and depressed:

Eat foods that are low in saturated fats and cholesterol (fruit, vegetables, cereals, pasta, low-fat dairy products, fish, poultry and lean meats). Limit salt intake by ignoring the saltshaker and avoiding highly salted, processed foods.

Cut calories if needed to attain and maintain your weight at recommended levels.

• Try to get adequate rest. The child's prayer that begins 'Now I lay me down to sleep' may be only wishful thinking for a lot of carers, but lack of sleep does play a part in depression. If you have sleepless nights and dreary days, consider hiring a helper for at least one of those nights so you can catch up.

There is sometimes a tendency on the part of carers to treat their loved ones as if they were physically ill with a disease that confines them to their homes; while this may be necessary during certain stages of Alzheimer's, it is usually not the case for all stages. Carers get to know the patterns of their loved ones; if they are content to sit and enjoy the scenery – as many are at certain stages – and others are available for assistance, there is no reason why carers need to give up many activities that give pleasure and foster health.

Carers need encouragement to get up, get out and get on with their lives, while including their loved ones in creative ways.

Keeping Mentally and Emotionally Balanced

There are a number of things we can do to help us keep our own minds engaged and our emotions on an even keel.

• Develop your sense of humour. One carer made the statement, 'I think people who don't have a sense of humour are the people that are really in trouble emotionally.' Do appreciate those lighter moments in your loved one's life. Try reminiscing about the good, fun and funny times you've had together.

Get acquainted with authors who know the human condition and who can write about it with humour and wisdom, such as Garrison Keillor, Pam Ayres and Joyce Grenfell. My own favourite British humorist is P. G. Wodehouse and I read my way though his many books a number of times during the years I spent caring for my mother. Subscribe to a magazine you enjoy. Read articles that can touch your heart and lift your spirits. Listen to books on tape or CD.

There's a proverb that says, 'Even in laughter the heart may ache.' We might also say that even in depression the heart may laugh. Without laughter, hearts can shrivel up and die.

• Maintain old hobbies and interests or develop new ones. Don't give up on the things you've enjoyed doing in the past – woodwork, reading, gardening, going to concerts, watching films at the cinema or at home. Incorporate your loved one into your activities, if you can, or hire help for an hour or a few hours each week (or find a volunteer) so you can get out and pursue your interests. That's a part of maintaining mental health. Both you and your loved one will be richer for it. During my own last year of caring I stopped working outside the home but ended up pursuing a dream of becoming a freelance writer. Staying at home, even with caring responsibilities, enabled me finally to do that. If you're not yet ready for retirement, expand your horizons and explore working-from-home options if that's where you need to be.

• A wheelchair can also be a worthwhile investment, not just for exercise but simply for going places. Even if your loved one is still able to walk well, wheelchairs can be useful for situations that require longer, more tiring walks.

With the aid of a wheelchair, I was able to take my mother Christmas shopping, to the zoo, to museums and galleries, and even camping at a state park equipped with caravans and nature trails designed for the disabled. For more information contact Holiday Care Service (see Appendix D for details).

Check with Social Services or Borough Surveyors about acquiring a disabled vehicle badge for the windscreen of your car. Generally only those people who have permanent and substantial difficulty in walking are eligible for concessionary parking under the 'Orange Badge scheme'. A doctor will have to sign a statement of need if the person does not already hold a mobility allowance. It's well worth the visit to obtain it.

• If music has been an important part of your loved one's life as well as your own, don't underestimate its value. Often the ability to play a musical instrument is still retained, though memory for other things is lost. Attend musical events together for as long as possible. Recent research indicates that music can also have a significant calming effect on people with dementia and may help to decrease symptoms of agitation.

• Maintain relationships with other people or develop new relationships. You may find it impossible to go out much, but you can invite people in. Don't feel they wouldn't want to come. Most people enjoy being invited out to eat. Suggest they bring a dish to share if your budget is tight. This may be a good way to get to know other carers, too, or even people in the neighbourhood; provide an evening 'out' for all concerned. One carer in our local support group whose husband had died continued to host annual picnics for the rest of us, including our relatives.

• If depression is a chronic or severe problem over which you seem to have little control, you may need to seek professional assistance. Your local GP will be one of the most important people for you to consult for an accurate diagnosis and assistance with an appropriate treatment plan; your GP may also be in the best position to make any needed referrals. There are many trained counsellors in private practice and local mental health clinics available with counsellors on hand. Members of the clergy can also be good sources of support and are usually well acquainted with depression. Sometimes medication may be needed as well as counselling. Signs and symptoms of a more severe depression can include:

generalized weakness/fatigue

uncontrollable or frequent episodes of crying

weight loss or, sometimes, weight gain

low blood pressure

headache or generalized aches and pains

constipation

sleep disturbances

memory lapses or confusion

symptoms of anxiety: tightness in the chest, stomach cramps, shaking, dizziness, a lump in the throat, sweating, diarrhoea, heart palpitations

excessive drinking

mood swings that range from euphoric to depressive

negative self-concept; low self-esteem

suicidal thoughts

Seeking Spiritual Support

Spiritual support for both you and your loved one can take many forms. One of the best support systems is a place of worship. My own experience of that is the local church.

Church, of all places, should be a place where you can take your loved one even in times of bizarre behaviour. Church families that are sensitive to the needs of memory-impaired people and their carers should be able to come up with some creative ways to help you both enjoy various aspects of the worship experience, whether on a Sunday morning or at various times throughout the week. If you don't find this to be true, talk to the priest, minister or vicar. You may have to make your needs known directly. You may also find you have to look around a bit for a church that meets your needs. Finding a good church can be a bit like finding a good home-care worker. Sooner or later, with persistence and prayer, you'll find the perfect match.

One church I know of gives carers a break each Sunday by offering free home care. People in the church take turns looking after a woman's husband, who is memory-impaired, so she can attend services. Another sponsors various carer support groups and offers training seminars on topics related to caring.

There is a movement called Parish Nursing that originated in the United States through the efforts of Granger Westberg and his daughter, Jill Westberg-McNamara, that has spread to many other countries, where nurses work in churches and often other faith communities like synagogues, to help coordinate care for members of the congregation. Some Parish Nurses lead carer support groups. Churches may also have health cabinets or wellness committees to foster health and wholeness. It is worth exploring to see if any places of worship near you have this particular service. (See Appendix D for more information on Parish Nursing.)

When I had got over my own anger at God and was looking for a church, I knew for certain when I had found the perfect match. This knowledge hit me one Sunday when, in the middle of the pastor's sermon, the congregation began singing 'Home on the Range'.

The reason for the song was an elderly man named George who suffered from dementia. Every Sunday the pastor's words would trigger something else in George's memory that related to a familiar song.

On this particular Sunday the pastor was talking about going to our heavenly home. The mention of 'home' was all George needed to break into a chorus of 'Home on the Range'. The pastor just smiled and encouraged the congregation to join in. So we all stood and sang. This, I thought, is a group of people who are comfortable with people with dementia!

Finding Joy in the Wilderness
Depression has often been called 'a wilderness experience'. Many people with Alzheimer's know this to be true. They become lost in

their own confusion and the tangled web of their minds. In the book *My Journey into Alzheimer's Disease*, Robert Davis, a Presbyterian minister diagnosed with Alzheimer's, wrote about one aspect of his own wilderness experience:

⏮ *I go to church services to worship God, but I cannot sing. I cannot join in the readings or prayers because my mind cannot do two things at once. Singing and group readings take several processes going on at once to listen to the others and pace my reading in time with theirs. Such a simple thing. But impossible for me now.*

Suddenly I stand out in the worship service, silent and continually confused during the time of hymn singing. I feel that my fellow worshippers are looking at me askance, wondering why I do not join in. My newfound paranoia also sets in, making me wonder if they think by my silence I am showing disapproval of the hymn, the church, the musicians, or the people around me. This time of joy has been changed into a time of frustration and anxiety.

Now I would like to come into the service late, after the singing of the first hymns or any responsive reading. However, out of propriety I do not. How I long to again sing my heart out and thus fully express my joy, but I cannot. The sorrow of this and this sense of loss fills me so much that often tears come to my eyes – tears that only compound my paranoia and my ever-present fears of what people are thinking.[2]

As carers we also experience the empty, barren wilderness as we gradually lose our loved one to a disease. As one carer asked, 'Where is the *essence* of my father?' The essence. Those indispensable, unique characteristics that make our loved one our loved one. Where are they? They're gradually lost with the progression of Alzheimer's disease, leaving us in a wilderness tinged with the memories of the past.

Elisabeth Elliot, in her book *Loneliness*, wrote the following: 'The wildernesses spoken of in the Bible were usually very barren places, but God can change that. He can make streams in the desert, springs in the valley, and furnish tables in the wilderness.'[3]

The streams and springs that God creates can turn our loneliness and depression into significantly different experiences. This often comes through friends, family and community carers who enter our world and give us help and opportunities for personal refreshment. Joy can come too as we are able to accept our circumstances and let God meet our own deepest needs for relationship.

PART FOUR

Saying Goodbye

Death is not darkness.
It is turning down the lamp
when dawn has broken.

RABINDRANATH TAGORE

Chapter Fifteen

The Difficult Decisions

A verse in the Bible reads: 'There is a time for everything, and a season for every activity under heaven' (Ecclesiastes 3:1).

Many will relinquish primary caring at home for a season of residential or nursing home care for their relative. For others, a season of caring at home will culminate in the death of a loved one. Neither change is easy; both bring a host of difficult decisions.

Knowing When to Give Up Caring at Home

It's time. Those two words are charged with conflicting emotions for carers who have finally made the decision to put their loved one in long-term care. The decision never comes easily but many carers know when *the time* is right.

⏮ *My husband had been crying a lot. He kept saying, 'Help me, help me, please help me,' over and over again. Nobody in the house was sleeping. Every day the furniture was turned upside down. He urinated in the middle of the kitchen. On weekends we just didn't bother with the house at all. People would come to visit and the chairs would be on top of the table. The couch was sometimes upside down. It was chaos.*

Then one day I got a call at work. My husband was at home, beating on the front door, crying and crying because he couldn't go out. One of the home-care helpers had called me, wondering what to do. A switch went on in my mind. I said to myself, 'It's time.'

The right time for long-term care is often related to the realization that we are no longer physically able to care for our loved one because of our own health problems.

⏮ *I've heard people say, 'I would never put my father or mother in a nursing home.' Well, I wouldn't have either if I could have handled him at home. But I couldn't. My mother couldn't. Physically we just couldn't handle it.*

You have to be practical. You have to realize when you simply can't cope any more – physically or emotionally. When you can no longer give the people you love most the care they should have, that's when you have to decide.

⏮ *I had help for eight hours a day prior to putting my husband in a nursing home. That still wasn't enough. I was up all night, every night. And I'm eighty-eight years old. It got to the point where I knew it was either him or me, and I knew I wasn't ready for a nursing home yet.*

Physical violence by our relative may be the last straw.

⏮ *One morning my husband hit me on the shoulder. He'd threatened me a good number of times, but he'd never actually done it before. It didn't really hurt, but it scared me.*

Just then the phone rang. It was my daughter. I was crying as I told her what had happened. She immediately called the social service worker who was already providing some home-care help for us.

The social worker came to see me that afternoon. That was a Monday. On Thursday my husband was admitted to the nursing home, one fairly close to our home.

I was glad he was going to that particular home. I'd visited it once before and liked it the best of any of them. That made the decision a little easier.

For others, safety may be the trigger issue – safety for our loved one and other family members.

⏮ *Daddy kept falling. We tried to prevent it, but the only way was to keep him restrained in a chair, and he fought that so. The other alternative was to sedate him, but then it*

---

was impossible for me to physically handle him. So we finally decided that, for his sake and mine, the nursing home was best.

◄◄ *The day my mother set the waste-paper basket on fire in the bedroom was the day we decided to do something. She just wasn't safe any more.*

So circumstances make us decide. Yet we still have to deal with our tangled emotions. And the predominant emotion is guilt.

Often, guilt surfaces because of others' attitudes.

◄◄ *There are so many people who think you put your parents in a nursing home because you want to get rid of them, that you don't want to be bothered, that you no longer care, that you don't appreciate what they did for you. They don't realize those are not the reasons at all.*

Fortunately, the initial guilt is often followed by the relief of knowing that, based on our situation, we have made the best decision for all concerned.

Don't be surprised, however, if ambivalent feelings remain.

◄◄ *Mum still feels guilty at times, but she knows Dad is getting good care.*

Mum really does worry about him. She prays for him every day. And I take her to see him once a week. She's prepared, if anything happens, to accept it.

We might be distressed if Dad were anywhere else but the home he's in. It's good, it's clean, and it's close. They're kind to him there. The doctor comes in every Friday and goes over his record and visits him. The doctor's on call if there's a problem.

All things considered, it's the best we could ask for.

◄◄ *There was a lot of guilt. The nursing home was the last place I ever wanted Daddy to go.*

When I went to visit him, I'd sit in the car and pray for strength to go in and go through all the conflicting emotions

I knew I'd have. I'd pray that I could act cheerful.

That first week I just wanted to pack Daddy up and take him home. I even thought of quitting my job to take care of him. But, even while I was thinking about it, I knew I couldn't. I knew it wasn't the best. For me. For my family. For Daddy.

⏮ *I still feel guilty whenever I visit my wife.*

The other night I went to see her and she hugged me and kissed me and seemed to know who I was. I cried. I couldn't help it.

But when she is not good and doesn't know me and doesn't pay any attention to me, I'm glad she's where she is.

So I'm up. And I'm down.

⏮ *I do feel guilty because I don't get to the nursing home as often as I used to. In the beginning I saw my father every other day. But then I suddenly realized there are other things that need to be taken care of.*

My mother, who's still at home, has needs too. Lots of them. I'm running her house too. She can live alone but she can't do her own cooking. I cook at home and make up frozen dinners for her.

I'm simply not always able to get up, get out and see my father every day.

We may wonder, 'Did I make the right decision?' But the day will come when we know for certain the answer is yes.

⏮ *In the beginning it was hard. Dad always wanted to come home with us. When it was time for us to leave, we'd say to the nurses, 'Please get Dad's attention.' And the nurses would try to distract him while we snuck out.*

Then one day when we were getting ready to go, Dad turned to us and said, 'You know, girls, this isn't a bad place. I rather like it. I think I'll buy it.'

> *All of a sudden, our guilt about institutionalization was gone.*

In the midst of this difficult decision making, some carers long for the good old days, an era when life was simple and families stayed together through thick and thin. Nancy Mace and Peter Rabins, in *The 36-Hour Day*, put the good old days in perspective:

◄◄ *We tend to think of the 'good old days' as a time when families took care of their elderly at home. In fact, in the past not many people lived long enough for their families to be faced with the burden of caring for a person with a demential illness. The people who did become old and sick were in their fifties and sixties and the sons and daughters who cared for them were considerably younger than you may be when your parent needs care in his seventies and eighties. Today many 'children' of an ailing parent are themselves in their sixties or seventies.*[1]

Times have changed. For today's families, the first goal is to support a loved one in whatever environment best meets his or her needs.

The second goal is to rid ourselves of the guilt that comes when nursing home placement is necessary. It may help to remember that nearly 70 per cent of nursing home beds are filled with people who suffer from Alzheimer's disease or a related dementia. We are not alone.

What Are the Options?
There are a number of options available for caring away from home on a long-term basis.

The residential care home
Residential homes are designed for people who don't require medical or nursing care, but who cannot live alone because of age, poor health or a chronic disability. Residents may be helped by care assistants with activities of daily living such as bathing, dressing, and

meal preparation and service. Not all homes will accept people with Alzheimer's, and some may take only a certain quota. On the other hand, more homes are now being opened exclusively for people with dementia. However, unless they are among the few homes 'dual registered' for both residential and nursing care, they may not be able to keep people when they become totally disabled and need more intensive nursing care. In practice, because residents are still able to receive the usual community nursing services and the care of their doctor, they may be able to remain in residential care without being transferred. Policies in homes may vary. Residential care homes also may provide short-term respite services for carers who need to get away for a holiday or may have work commitments that require travel (see Chapter Eleven).

A social worker may help you to obtain a place for your relative in a local-authority-run or private residential home. Prior to any placement you will be asked to consent to an assessment of need in order to determine the best placement option for your loved one. If you ask in advance, it may be possible for your loved one to have a trial stay or perhaps to visit on a day basis. Homes too will need to do an assessment to make sure they are able to provide the appropriate level of care for your loved one. They have a right to refuse if they believe they are not able to meet your loved one's needs; if a person with dementia also develops behaviours that can be more difficult to manage once they are in a residential home, families may be consulted about the need to explore different housing options where more supervision is available. Some homes may also have waiting lists, so if you have a particular home in mind you might consider placing your loved one on the list. If you are exploring options, consider using a checklist of criteria. Some guidelines and resources are included in Appendix A.

The same is true of profit-making private residential homes and non-profit-making voluntary homes. Size and type of accommodation and standards of care vary tremendously and it is impossible to make generalizations. Check that the home is registered with the local authority and inspected regularly (a legal requirement). Talk with other carers and with groups such as Age Concern if you are in any doubt. Many people prefer residential care initially because of the homey atmosphere and personal attention offered, but nursing home placement provides a higher level of care when people need more assistance with all the activities of daily living.

Hospital care

People with Alzheimer's may be placed in the older person wards of general hospitals or in mental health settings. Generally, when people with Alzheimer's are hospitalized it is not because of Alzheimer's but for some other reason such as a fracture following a fall or pneumonia. This can be a good time though for further assessment related to dementia. The National Health Service covers hospital care initially; it is paid for through the National Insurance Contributions of people who are employed, so it is actually an earned benefit rather than a free service. Your loved one's National Insurance Pension may be reduced after the first eight weeks as a contribution to care. Short hospital stays are the norm today with more and more services available in the community for follow-up care at home or in other settings such as nursing homes.

Nursing homes

There are various types of nursing home. Most are privately run: some are run by voluntary or charitable organizations, and some are local authority or council-run through Social Services. Some privately run homes are considered *proprietary*, which means they expect to make a profit. Others are *non-proprietary*, or non-profit. Nursing care is provided by qualified staff twenty-four hours a day, including qualified professional nurses and trained staff who care for personal needs. Residents in nursing homes require more assistance with activities of daily living than those in residential care and may also need to be assisted with feeding and toileting. There is some level of doctor coverage for all nursing homes, though doctors do not generally work in the homes. Specialists from the hospital may be called in if there is a need indicated by the GP. Usually a resident is monitored by their own GP or would have the opportunity to change to a more local practice for physician coverage if needed. Appendix A includes more information on nursing home inspections and how to obtain inspection reports.

Special care/Dementia units

Some hospitals and nursing homes have special-care units for people with dementia. These are usually units that allow people to freely wander in a supervised environment. I have worked on a number of these units in the United States that were located in nursing homes and found them to be particularly suited to the person with Alzheimer's. They are generally staffed by nurses and others who have special training and who also acquire training by working exclusively in one environment. The Alzheimer's Society and your Alzheimer's local support group should be good sources for specific information.

Quality varies from home to home and has little to do with a home's profit or non-profit status. From my own experience, quality of care depends on the training and attitudes of the personnel.

Looking for a Long-term Care Facility

There are many things to consider when looking for a suitable home away from home for your relative. The following points may help to make things easier:

• Talk to other carers who have placed loved ones with Alzheimer's in alternative living situations. How did they choose that particular home? Are they happy or unhappy with it? Why?

• Seek out nurses, social workers or others in your community who work with the elderly, specifically people with Alzheimer's and other types of dementia. Ask what's available in the area.

• Keep your own limitations and the concerns of your family in mind. For instance, there may be an excellent home several hours away that has a special unit for people with Alzheimer's. Is this an option? Would visitation by family and friends still be possible?

• Meet with your relative's GP. It's good to have a doctor involved early in the planning process, for information and support. Also, a doctor's referral will usually be needed for an assessment prior to admission to a nursing home.

Unfortunately, many carers shop for a nursing home as they shop for Christmas presents. At the last minute.

This is unwise. Plan ahead. This will enable you to choose the home best suited to your relative's personality and needs. If your relative always attended church, for example, and was active in a weekly Bible study, consider a home that has a wider range of religious activities. Don't wait for a crisis and then expect a bed to be available. Chances are, it won't.

Reasons for advance planning include the following:

Waiting lists

Most homes in the UK have them. Even if you're unsure about placement, it's wise to fill out an application at a number of homes. (You can always say no if you are called and are not ready to place. Just ask the home to call you again in the future.) With hospitals discharging patients quicker and sicker, some homes are more likely to admit directly from the hospital itself. Your loved one may not be able to go to a nursing home of your choice if they are admitted from the hospital and the waiting list at that particular home is long.

Some homes limit the number of people they will admit with dementia. In this case, it's essential that your loved one be placed on a waiting list.

Legal loose ends

There's always a need to explore legal issues related to residential and nursing home placement. It takes time to tie up loose ends. Don't shortchange yourself.

Additional Criteria and Resources

The Brief Care Home Guide and *The Complete Care Home Guide* are very helpful resources for carers that cover a wide range of topics on caring options and costs. They can both be downloaded from websites or ordered from Counsel and Care, a national charity supporting older people, their families and carers.[2] The Alzheimer's Society also has a number of fact sheets available on all aspects of alternative care, including residential and nursing home care. It is well worth exploring these websites as a carer.

In addition to using a guide or checklist, evaluate a nursing home or any other similar facility using your own common sense and common *senses*. Visit several facilities. Planned visits with the nursing home social workers and/or nursing home administrators are essential, but you may also want to arrive unexpectedly, too. Talk with some of the residents and their families. Observe the residents involved in activities, both social and health related. Watch the nursing home staff at work. Pay attention to first impressions and to what your senses are telling you.

What do you *feel*? Does the place *feel* like a home or an institution? Even in very large homes, caring, compassionate, non-institutional attitudes will show – if the staff have them.

What do you *see*? The best homes combine good nursing care with a homelike atmosphere. Are individual rooms cheerful, with pictures on the wall and mementoes from home? Are the majority of residents out of bed, dressed for the day, and well groomed? Do most appear alert? *Alert* does not necessarily mean 'oriented'. It has more to do with wakefulness. If the majority of residents are not alert, it may be a sign of inappropriate medication or even of boredom if there are few activities in the home.

Do the nursing assistants (the people doing most of the hands-on care) look frenzied and frazzled or do they appear relatively calm and relaxed? Ask about the aide-to-resident ratio; you'll want to know if the home is adequately staffed.

What do you *hear*? Pay attention to what people are saying and their tone of voice. Do the staff talk to the residents? What do they talk about? Do they speak to them with dignity and respect?

Don't be unduly upset if you hear residents shout or scream at times. Bath and shower times are prime occasions for this; confused residents may resent this intrusion or be frightened.

What do you *smell*? It's not possible to have a completely odour-free environment in a nursing home. You may note the smell of urine or stool coming from a room or two as you walk down the corridor. This should be an exception rather than the rule. If there is a pervasive odour of urine or some other unpleasant smell, ask why. You should also see housekeeping staff mopping and damp dusting.

Ask the nursing director what kind of training staff receive. Extensive training of all nursing personnel should be a requirement; often basic training is done prior to being hired through other educational facilities. Homes should have an orientation period for all staff that includes: an overview of residents' rights; issues related to resident abuse, mistreatment and neglect; the problems of ageing; fire safety for staff and residents; and training in the proper methods of lifting and moving residents. You may ask to see a copy of the orientation programme. This will be readily available in most nursing homes. Feel free to ask questions about any of these issues.

How Do I Pay the Bills?

One of the first questions a nursing home will ask the family of a prospective resident is, 'Who will pay the bill?' Nursing homes usually aren't cheap. But their cost covers nutritious meals, your relative's share of the rent and utilities, and medical and nursing care that involves many trained personnel. An initial comprehensive social service assessment prior to placement should include an evaluation by a case manager to determine the actual type and level of care needed, a financial assessment to determine your loved one's and/or your contribution to the care required, and an assessment as to what specific nursing care might be required. The NHS does currently pay for services by nurses in nursing homes.

Different facilities have different fee structures. Rates will also vary depending on the type of room a person has; for example, private, or shared with one or more other residents. Some homes will only accept residents who are paying privately while others may accept only residents whose care is covered by the NHS; some accept both. Financial assessments are required for you to receive any type of government funding. Homes are required to give you written information about costs and you should feel free to ask questions if any information is unclear. Paying for alternative care can be handled in a variety of ways, including the following:

Private funds

Some families are able to pay for nursing home care privately, though not necessarily for ever. Costs will vary and may increase annually. You should consider a financial assessment even if you are paying privately, as some costs may be covered for your loved one by government funding.

Spouses, children and other responsible parties will need to consult with a solicitor about their own financial liability and other issues of concern. For example, are you legally and financially responsible for a parent in a nursing home? For all or part of their care? Talk with the nursing home social worker, but don't sign anything until you've also checked with your own financial adviser.

Benefits

Given the high cost of nursing care, it is vital to be aware of any benefits to which you or your relative are entitled. These include invalidity benefit (payable to a person incapable of work, up until retirement age) and the retirement pension. Widow's benefits include an initial lump sum, the widowed mother's allowance and the widow's pension (for those with no dependent children). Varying criteria apply.

Income Support and/or housing benefit may also be claimed by those in residential or nursing homes, to help with fees.

No benefits are paid automatically and a written claim must be made, in some cases with medical evidence. Claim forms are available from local post offices, Department of Social Security Offices and

Citizens Advice Centres, and specialist advice can be obtained from the Alzheimer's Society or Age Concern. In some UK countries (this includes England, Wales and Northern Ireland but not Scotland) the person with dementia who has assets over a certain amount will be required to contribute some of those assets to fund part of the cost of care. This could mean the sale of a family home for a person who lives alone, though this would not be required if a spouse is living there and there may be other exceptions for other dependants or carers.

Insurance and pensions

Private health insurance and certain life insurance and pension plans may also cover some nursing home costs. Some plans are excellent, while others pay negligible amounts for custodial-type care. Talk directly with your insurance agent or a company representative about available benefits.

Ex-armed services benefits

If your loved one was a member of the armed services, enquire about benefits. It is also worth finding out about any ex-armed services nursing homes in your area; speak with them directly about medical and financial eligibility. The Ex-Services Homes Referral Agency (ESHRA) has a database of all nursing, convalescent and respite care homes for veterans in the UK.[3]

Making That Difficult Decision

As you weigh the pros and cons of placement, consider the following issues and questions. Your responses should help you make a wise and appropriate decision based on your loved one's needs and the needs of your family.

• *Health.* Can you continue to care for your loved one at home without jeopardizing your own mental, emotional and physical health? What about the health of other family members? Is the care you're able to provide keeping your relative as healthy as possible – or is ill health increasing in frequency, duration or intensity?

- *Safety*. Can you continue to provide a safe environment, or are accidents increasingly beyond your control? Is the safety of the rest of the family at risk if your relative remains at home?

- *Support*. Do you have enough support from family, friends and community services to handle increasing care needs? Is the help you need (or will need) affordable as well as available?

Placing my own mother in a nursing home was not an easy decision for me. I was one of those people who had always told myself, 'I'll never do it.' But then, one day, I did, just like other carers have done. Health, safety and support were all factors in making the decision. It seemed that Mum and I were spending more and more time on the floor; she was no longer able to walk as the Alzheimer's progressed into the final stages, and transfers from chair to bed or wheelchair to car were becoming increasingly difficult. Safety for both of us was an issue, coupled with dwindling finances and a decision I had made to move to another city to continue my education. Mum's unexpected trip to the hospital for a condition unrelated to her Alzheimer's was the trigger event that convinced me that 'now was the time'. Friends and relatives were supportive, realizing better than I that home care was not really providing the best for her, no matter how well I thought I was coping.

Continuing to Care

You can still care for a loved one in practical ways after he or she moves to a nursing home or hospital. Relinquishment does not mean abandonment. In fact, a good home will welcome any support you can offer. This includes visits as well as helpful hints – drawn from your years of experience – about caring for your relative.

- People who are confused do better in familiar surroundings. Suggest arranging the furniture as it was at home, if this is possible. Some homes will even allow you to bring in familiar furniture. Also bring pictures, photographs and, of course, your relative's favourite clothes.

• It's generally good to be with your loved one on the day of admission, though situations may differ. You won't necessarily need to stay all day, but several hours will be helpful for the initial transition. Take someone with you for support – another family member or a best friend. Don't assume loved ones won't adjust. Sometimes they settle in immediately; if they no longer recognize familiar faces, everyone may be family to them.

• Before or on the day of admission the nurse will want to know more about your loved one's background. This is called 'taking a social history'. As a nurse, I find social histories to be vitally important. The history might include the type of work your loved one used to do, places of employment, special hobbies and interests, information about children and grandchildren (including names and addresses), religious affiliation and involvement, languages spoken, and so on. Unfortunately, on some charts the information is very sparse, either because there is no family to give it or because families feel the information is too personal.

The activities department of the home can use this information to plan a programme suited to your loved one's needs. For example, if your relative was very active in church, provisions can be made for attending worship services and special religious services in the home. Other activities might include social hours, in-house movies, bingo or baking. A person with Alzheimer's may not be able to participate actively in these activities but they may enjoy socializing in a group.

A social history can also be helpful for the nursing assistants caring for your loved one. Knowing something about your loved one's interests and occupation can provide a point of contact for conversation or provide the carers with something to talk about.

Anne Evans and John Smith exemplify the value of a detailed social history. Anne Evans was a resident in the early stages of Alzheimer's who had been very depressed. I attended one of the care conferences when the staff talked about possible reasons for her depression and suggested ways to cheer her up. Leafing through her social history, I noticed that she had been an avid golfer. I went home that night, wrapped up a new package of golf balls and brought it in the next day. Anne and I unwrapped the package together. This small action didn't cure her depression, but it brightened her day and provided a point of contact. She enjoyed talking about this past interest, and that opened the door for discussing those interests as well as other more immediate concerns.

John Smith was a resident who was in the advanced stages of dementia with markedly depressed consciousness. A nursing assistant told me, 'I always turn his radio to a classical music station when I take care of him. One of his relatives told me he played the violin and was in an orchestra when he was younger.' That information wasn't part of Mr Smith's social history. I added a note to the chart and we put a sign on the radio about keeping it tuned to a particular station.

These pieces of helpful information can easily be forgotten in the busyness of a loved one's admission. Feel free, though, to pass them along (preferably in writing) at any time, so they can be shared with staff members and benefit your loved one.

• Continuing to visit is important. Some people visit daily, others weekly, others less frequently. There is no right or wrong schedule. Feel your way into a visitation schedule that meets the needs of everyone involved.

Visiting doesn't always have to be in the home. You may want to take your loved one out: go to a restaurant, have a picnic in the park, go shopping or attend church. Going back to a previous home may or may not be an option to consider. Some people easily adjust to this; but others want to stay at home once they get there. Some people with Alzheimer's experience increased stress related to outings and home visits and may actually be better off remaining in the home; don't feel guilty if this is the case, even on holidays that are normally family occasions. The staff will be honest with you if you ask them about how your loved one readjusts to the nursing home routine after a home visit.

When you do visit, use the time to care for your loved one in practical ways. Give a manicure, go for a walk or a wheelchair ride, assist with feeding at mealtimes (unless nursing home policy prohibits this). Actually doing something physical may help you feel better about the visit. If your loved one has always enjoyed literature, spend time reading to them.

Continuing-care Issues

Once your loved one settles in, concerns will continue to arise. Talk to the charge nurse, social worker or director of nursing about any problems. Remember, though, that some things will be done very differently than they were at home. The use of restraints of some type (waist or vest) was quite common in nursing homes and hospitals in the United States, based on the belief that they would protect the person from falling out of bed or out of a chair and prevent injury. As noted earlier, restraints are rarely used today as research indicates that injuries sustained by people falling who have been restrained may be more severe than injuries sustained by those who have not been restrained. In residential and nursing homes there will be alternative means to prevent people with dementia from wandering out of the home, such as special chairs, bed alarms and bracelets that might set off an alarm if a person tries to exit the facility. If you have any questions about the type or quality of care given, talk to the people in charge. Let your concerns be known.

• Take advantage of planned activities, such as nursing home picnics or holiday events, which enhance staff and family relationships. This can be a less stressful time to get to know the staff more personally. Nursing homes truly are extended families in many ways. These types of activities, when everyone is really enjoying each other's company, can help you see the home as a caring community of friends.

• Inevitably, questions arise concerning care should a loved one stop breathing. What should be done? Should he or she be resuscitated?

In some facilities all staff are trained in CPR (cardiopulmonary resuscitation) and would be expected to try to revive any resident suffering a cardiac or respiratory arrest. In other homes, staff would immediately call an ambulance. The ambulance team might then attempt to resuscitate. This would not be done, however, for any resident who has a DNR (do not resuscitate) order. In cases where a resident is considered terminally ill or is in the more advanced stages of Alzheimer's, DNR orders would generally apply as well. The best policy is to discuss in advance what measures should be taken in case of emergency; generally this is done with the physician, nursing staff and/or social worker. This is an important area to discuss with family members prior to nursing home placement. Also, talk with the nurse in the home to find out if the home can provide end-of-life care that is supportive rather than transferring people to the hospital. Supportive care in one's own home or in a long-term care facility can generally provide a quieter atmosphere and one that is more comfortable for the person and their relatives at the end of life.

• Finally, stay in tune with your feelings. Be involved in a support group. Some nursing homes have support groups that regularly meet in the home. Ask about them.

Guilt, anger and depression do not automatically disappear the day you walk through the nursing home door, or the day you walk out and leave your loved one behind. But we can deal with all these emotions the same way we dealt with them when our loved ones were at home: with support from others, help from God and the understanding that what we're experiencing is normal. We *will* survive.

The Post-mortem and After

Without a post-mortem of brain tissue, doctors may be reluctant to cite Alzheimer's disease as the cause of death, even if your loved one exhibited all the classic signs and symptoms. Feelings and beliefs about the post-mortem, however, can vary widely.

◄◄ *My grandfather said, 'No post-mortem. Your grandmother's been through enough hurt already. We don't need to do that to her.'*

◄◄ *I've made plans for my father's brain tissue to be donated for research. As a matter of fact, I have a post-mortem file.*

When I left for holiday recently I told a friend, 'Here's the file. If anything happens to Dad, get the file to my brother. He'll have to act immediately.'

I have the materials filed both in the nursing home and at the hospital where Dad's doctor practices, so they'll know this is what we want.

It's a very difficult thing to plan. Just the thought of what they'll have to do hurts me terribly. But if it can help future victims – if it can help future generations of our own family – it will be worth the tears.

◄◄ *When I'm alone, bored and the weather's nasty, I think about Mum's death and the post-mortem. I know it had to be done.*

There was the chance that they would find something in her brain that would give them a clue as to what really goes wrong. And I know my mother would have said, 'Do it, if it's going to help someone else.'

◄◄ *I was planning on having a post-mortem autopsy done right up until the time of my mother's death; then I changed my mind at the last minute. I thought particularly about my mum and her feelings about personal privacy.*

I felt guilty about my decision at first but I don't any more. I don't see this as a moral issue or an issue of right or wrong, but as a personal one that every relative makes based on their own particular circumstances.

Requesting a post-mortem examination (or autopsy) of the brain and arranging the donation of brain tissue is a final step many carers decide to take, for a number of reasons.

Post-mortems conclusively confirm or deny the presence of Alzheimer's disease

During an autopsy, the pathologist microscopically examines sections of the brain. If Alzheimer's was present, there will be plaques and tangles, the disease's main characteristics. This is how Alzheimer's was believed to be originally diagnosed.

If Alzheimer's was the cause of the dementia, treatment for symptomatic relatives may be possible. Family members could then take advantage of experimental drug research and medical advances if diagnosed early.

Families will also want to know if plaques and tangles are absent. For people worried about the disease's genetic possibilities, such news can offer relief.

The only other test that can conclusively confirm or deny Alzheimer's is a brain biopsy, performed while the patient is alive, but these are rarely done due to the very high risk of complications.

The clinical diagnosis of Alzheimer's disease made while a person is living can be inaccurate, no matter how much testing is done. Only brain autopsies after death can provide conclusive evidence.

Post-mortems contribute to Alzheimer's research

Studying the living brain is difficult. Unlike other major organs, the brain is not easily probed. It's encased in a bony 'safe' designed to protect it from infection and trauma.

The brain also has the added protection of a special membrane called the blood-brain barrier, which prevents undesirable chemicals from entering the brain. This protective sheath makes it equally difficult to withdraw any foreign chemicals from living brain tissue, chemicals that might give clues to Alzheimer's cause.

Alzheimer's is a uniquely human disease that affects our thoughts, emotions, personality and will, but researchers have found animals like mice useful in recent years to study some important aspects of Alzheimer's; for example, its molecular biology and potential drug treatments. In the UK, the Alzheimer's Research Trust supports research using animal models.

Post-mortems help generate funding for research

Funding for research for any disease is based largely on its prevalence. In the case of Alzheimer's, it's especially important that accurate statistics are gathered.

These factors highlight the importance of brain tissue research. A cure is unlikely unless a cause is discovered, and no cause will be discovered without continuing exploration into the abnormalities of autopsied human brain cells.

Consenting to a Post-mortem Brain Autopsy

The decision to have a post-mortem done in which the brain is specifically autopsied should not be left to the emotion-laden days surrounding the death of a loved one. A sudden, unexpected death could eliminate the opportunity for an autopsy because of the necessary medical and legal requirements. As prepared as I thought I was, this happened with my own mother. I had moved to another part of the state and was in the process of obtaining autopsy forms and trying to arrange for nursing home placement in the new area for my mother when the call came from the nursing home that Mum's condition had changed for the worse. Foresight and planning are essential well before a crisis hits.

A great deal of information, guidance and support is needed before a decision for a post-mortem can be made. Help is available from a number of sources:

• Start with your local support group. Ask others in the group if they have gone through this process. Have a speaker on the subject come to a meeting and discuss the regulations that apply to your community.

• Think through the reasons for a post-mortem and weigh the pros and cons. You or your relative may have religious objections. Talk to your pastor, priest or rabbi if this is a concern for you.

You may feel that your loved one's body will be desecrated or treated with disrespect. Rest assured that a brain autopsy causes no disfigurement to a person's face or body. There is no reason why, following an autopsy, you cannot have an open-casket viewing or funeral.

• Many research projects related to dementia – for example, those for experimental medications – see great value in post-mortem brain examinations and may request permission from persons with dementia whom they are studying and their carers. When death does occur in the future the researchers would have access to this information for further study.

• Discuss the decision with family members. If there is a surviving spouse, the ultimate decision rests with him or her. Still, it is good to agree as a family – and all family members will have an opinion on the subject, coloured by their emotions, knowledge of what's involved and beliefs about what their relative would have wanted, which is a legitimate concern.

• Send for the information sheet on Brain Tissue Donations from the Alzheimer's Society. As well as suggestions for practical arrangements, this includes a list of research centres that would be grateful for the donation of post-mortem material for further study.

Making Medical Arrangements

Make sure that you speak to your relative's doctor and the staff of the nursing home to find out what arrangements will be needed for a brain autopsy. You may need to make special provisions in case your loved one should die on a weekend or on holiday, and there may be a time limit involved.

If you have decided on brain tissue donation, contact the nearest research centre in good time, for the necessary information. Forms will need to be filled in and plans made with the local pathologist. In some cases there will be costs for transportation to the research centre.

Remember also that the funeral director must be involved and aware of your wishes. The body should not be embalmed before the brain is removed.

Knowing the Truth

Several months after an autopsy you or your doctor should receive a written, detailed explanation of the autopsy results from the neuropathologist who conducted the autopsy. This will include a diagnosis based on both large-scale and microscopic findings.

Consenting to a post-mortem is never a painless decision for anyone who is a carer and carers should not feel guilty if they decide against this procedure. After all the suffering our loved one has experienced, we may feel he or she is entitled to rest in peace. But if we see the autopsy as an aid to research and as the ultimate diagnostic test for a disease that, someday, may be arrested, prevented and cured, it becomes a painful decision that offers promise. For us, our loved ones and our families, the battle may soon be over. For millions of others, it has only just begun. The information gained from our relative's post-mortem may be the vital link in the chain that will one day reveal the true cause of this devastating disease.

Chapter Sixteen

Blowing Out the Candle

Muriel sat at the kitchen table. The wick in the paraffin lamp flared, casting a warm glow over the chilled room. The storm had abated but the electricity was still out. Muriel sat, stared at the flame, and thought about her mother's death several days earlier.

Her mother's death had been a lot like that flickering wick. A lot like the dimly burning candle that sat on the mantelpiece in the dining room.

Death had not come easily for Ruth. Neither had life. She had always worked so hard. Worked hard raising three children. Worked hard on the farm with her husband. And when she developed Alzheimer's, Ruth worked incredibly hard, for many years, to cover it up.

Then Ruth had died hard – labouring to breathe, to stay alive, to keep the fire of life burning.

Muriel remembered that some of her friends, children of parents with Alzheimer's, said death was a relief. It was a release from years of suffering. Muriel wasn't so sure. It didn't seem like that for her mother. What was death really like? What would it be like for her? Was it a foe to be fought or a friend to be welcomed?

Muriel lowered the wick in the paraffin lamp and watched as the smoke curled around inside the glass globe. She walked over to the candle on the mantelpiece above the fireplace. One blow. Two. A third finally snuffed the flame.

Just like Mum, thought Muriel. Just like most of us – working hard to keep our candle burning.

Caring for the Dying

For some loved ones, death will come quietly, quickly. For others it will come only with more struggles, more suffering. The way of death is not something we can explain or understand. We can merely wait, prepare and pray that we can make it a little easier for our loved ones and ourselves.

When the nursing home called me about a change in my mother's condition, it was the week before Easter. I made the four-hour trip out to see her and planned to go with her to the hospital for a series of tests related to gastrointestinal bleeding, which she had developed. But just prior to her scheduled tests, Mum's condition deteriorated and it was soon apparent to all concerned that the primary concern was now related to her breathing.

I was faced with a decision. My mother's doctor gave me the options: acute hospital care or comfort care at the nursing home with a staff well equipped to keep my mother as pain-free and comfortable as possible. I chose the latter course of action and spent the next three days (and most of the evenings and nights) sitting at her bedside, holding her hand, and assisting the nurses and aides with her personal care. When death came, it was not without a struggle, for both of us; but it came as I would have hoped it would. Mum was not alone. It was clearly evident from the tears of the nursing assistants that I was not the only 'family member' who had loved her.

Caring for someone approaching the final days of life either at home or in a nursing facility is not very different from caring for any other very ill person. If your loved one is confined to a bed and needs total care for a lengthy period, your goals are to keep him or her comfortably positioned, clean, dry and as pain-free as possible.

• Keep the room well aired and well lit. Good ventilation makes breathing easier and provides a more pleasant environment for you to work in. A dark room can be a frightening place for someone who is dying, especially someone with Alzheimer's.

• Because of poor circulation, your loved one may feel cold. This will be especially noticeable in the hands and feet. Lightweight blankets and duvets will help.

• Skin care is vitally important as poor circulation and inadequate nutrition take their toll on the body's ability to nourish cells. Turn your loved one frequently, at least every two hours. Give soothing back massages. Pay special attention to the skin over any bony prominences such as the hips, the bottom of the spine, heels, elbows, shoulders, and even the back of the head and the ears. Consider obtaining a water, air, gel or foam mattress for the bed to prevent skin breakdown.

• Heels and elbows can be padded and wrapped with gauze if your loved one thrashes against side rails. Sheepskin and foam slippers are also available.

• Position extra pillows to increase comfort and decrease pressure on legs and arms.

• Bowel and bladder control will diminish even more until there is total incontinence. Keep your loved one as clean and dry as possible. A laundry service, if available, will help greatly.

A catheter, which may be inserted by a district nurse with a doctor's order, may help remove urine from the bladder. This can easily be maintained at home, provided your loved one is relatively still and doesn't pull it out.

• Keeping your loved one hydrated and nourished will become increasingly difficult. The ability to swallow may eventually be lost altogether. In the meantime, provide favourite foods that are high in calories.

When swallowing becomes more difficult, offer puddings, yoghurt, pureed fruits and ice cream. Sometimes milk products and citrus fruit juices will increase mucus production and cause problems. If this is the case, switch to non-dairy products and juices, such as apple and grape. Thickeners are available for juices and can even be put in water to make swallowing easier. A district nurse should be able to help you obtain these. Consult your local chemist.

• Ice cubes may be welcome if sucking can be done without danger of choking. When swallowing becomes more of a problem, moisten a face-cloth in iced water and let your loved one suck on it.

• Good mouth care is essential. Your loved one will probably breathe through the mouth, and the jaw will sag. The mouth can become very dry and uncomfortable as a result. Frequent liquids can help, but also consider purchasing some mouth swabs. Use them often.

• Placing a very light layer of petroleum jelly on lips and around nasal passages may help prevent cracking.

• If your loved one is bothered by an excessive amount of mucus build-up in the mouth, you may want to rent a suction machine. You can hire an in-home nurse to operate this, or ask for instruction from a district nurse on how to use it yourself.

• A sitting or semi-sitting position is best for eating and can help prevent choking. (Renting or borrowing an adjustable hospital bed will make this more practical. Special chairs are also available for a reclined and comfortable sitting position.)

One of the best investments you can make at any time during your loved one's illness is a good nurse's-aide or nursing-assistant manual. Such manuals offer hundreds of additional tips on how to feed, position, bathe, toilet and otherwise meet the physical needs of people who are ill. Titles may change from year to year; enquire through a nursing home or home nursing agency about what book they use and order one through them, or from the publisher, any bookstore or on-line. Good quality and up-to-date books are often available used and can be very economical.

Should terminal care prove overwhelming for you, consider getting outside assistance through a local nursing agency or hospice programme. The latter features professional carers and volunteers who emphasize pain control and meeting the physical, emotional and spiritual needs of patient and carer, in as natural an environment as possible. Some agencies offer sliding-fee scales based on ability to pay. In some areas a Terminal Care Service may be available to assist carers in nursing those who are dying at home. Some nursing homes also provide hospice-type care with trained hospice nurses for the terminally ill during the last weeks of their life; this may be available in your area.

Emotional and Spiritual Support

'What is it about death that makes you afraid?' I once asked an elderly woman in a nursing home.

'The dying part,' she replied.

'But what about the dying part?' I asked, hoping she'd be more specific.

'The part about dying alone,' she said.

We can provide emotional and spiritual support for loved ones simply by being with them. We can hold their hands, offer back rubs and remind them that we love them. We can assure them that they won't need to fear the dying part; they won't be abandoned. They are not alone.

We can also pray for our loved ones, asking God to ease their last days and make the transition from this life to the next an easier one.

I once led weekly Bible studies in a nursing home for a small group of residents with Alzheimer's. Our favourite passage, and one we read frequently, was Psalm 23. According to the writer of this psalm, death does not have to be a lonely experience. There is someone to walk through the valley of the shadow of death with us. Remind your loved one of this; remind yourself.

Brightly Burning Wicks

A number of years before my mother's death, I broke her walking stick. It happened the morning I was late for work because the helper I had hired was late. 'My car broke down,' she said on the phone. 'I'll be there when I can.'

Frustration. I was supposed to be covering for a sick co-worker at the office. I had to get there as soon as possible.

My mother wasn't helping. When I tried to get her out of bed, she resisted. When I finally got her on her feet, she decided to sit down on the floor. That's when she began striking my legs with her stick. She didn't hit me hard, but I lost control. I grabbed the stick and banged it against the floor. The walking stick, old and fragile, snapped in two. It lay broken on the floor beside my mother.

I felt shame and horror. My first thought was, What if that had been my mother? Would anger or frustration ever make me treat her like that walking stick?

Mum brought me back to the present. She was still sitting on the floor. But now she was laughing. I sat down beside her, put my arms around her and laughed too. I laughed until I cried.

That night I read this verse from the book of Isaiah: 'A bruised reed he will not break, and a dimly burning wick he will not quench.' That struck a nerve. At times, I felt like a bruised reed, bruised and battered in the battle against Alzheimer's.

My mother was a bruised reed, too, a fragile person incapable of caring for herself or understanding what was happening. A person who needed to be cared for gently – with love, laughter and, occasionally, tears.

But for me the verse in Isaiah held a promise from God. Neither of us would be broken. Neither of us had to walk through life alone, despite the suffering and confusion. God promised to hold our hands. He would also *stay* my hand and give me patience as a carer.

Later, I hauled the broken stick out of the rubbish and put it in the linen cupboard. And now, years later, it still rests on a shelf in a cupboard where I currently live with my husband and stepson, serving as a reminder for me to be gentle with those whose lives are flickering in the darkness.

It reminds me, too, that we are not alone.

Part Four: Saying Goodbye

Appendix A

Evaluating Long-term Care Options

There are many resources available to carers about long-term care options such as nursing homes, care homes and residential care facilities. The following are some of the most easily accessible websites with further information. See Appendix D for additional agencies and organizations.

The Alzheimer's Disease International website has very helpful information on choosing a nursing home or other facility. See the following link that also includes links to various Alzheimer's associations throughout the world: http://www.alz.co.uk/carers/help. html

The Commission for Social Care Inspection is an organization that inspects and reports on care services and councils. On their website you can find information about various care services and homes, such as free inspection reports and checklists including questions to ask when visiting a care home. They have information on getting a care assessment from your council and on different types of care and payment options. See: http://www.csci.org.uk/

Careuk.net, an NHFA website, aims to point individuals to some of the numerous sources of support, advice and information available throughout the UK. Their website includes a downloadable long-term care guide. This website has very useful information about residential and nursing home care and payment issues in particular. See: http://www.careuk.net/Page_NHFABestPractice.asp

Checklist for Evaluating a Nursing Home

1. Does the home have a current licence from the local health authority?

2. Does the home provide special services, such as a specific diet or therapy, which the patient needs?

PHYSICAL CONSIDERATIONS

3. Locations
    a pleasing to the patient?
    b convenient to a doctor?
    c convenient for frequent visits?

4. Accident prevention
    a well-lit inside?
    b free of hazards underfoot?
    c handrails in hallways and bathrooms?

5. Fire safety
    a meets fire regulations?
    b exits clearly marked and unobstructed?
    c written emergency-evacuation plan?
    d frequent fire drills?
    e exit doors not locked on the inside?
    f stairways enclosed and doors to stairways kept closed?

6. Bedrooms
    a open onto a hall?
    b windows?
    c acceptable number of beds per room?
    d easy access to each bed?
    e nurse-call bell by each bed?
    f fresh drinking water available?
    g at least one comfortable chair per person?
    h reading lights?

   i wardrobe and drawers?

   j room for a wheelchair to manoeuvre?

   k care exercised when selecting room-mates?

7. Cleanliness

   a generally clean, even though it may have a lived-in look?

   b free of unpleasant odours?

   c incontinent patients given prompt attention?

8. Vestibule

   a welcoming atmosphere?

   b if also a lounge, is it being used by residents?

   c furniture attractive and comfortable?

   d plants and flowers?

   e certificates and licences on display?

9. Hallways

   a large enough for two wheelchairs to pass with ease?

   b handrails on the sides?

10. Dining room

   a attractive and inviting?

   b comfortable chairs and tables?

   c easy to move around in?

   d tables convenient for those in wheelchairs?

   e food tasty and attractively served?

   f meals match the posted menu?

   g those needing help receiving it?

11. Kitchen

   a food preparation, dishwashing and rubbish areas separated?

   b food needing refrigeration not standing on counters?

   c kitchen help observing hygiene rules?

12. Activity rooms

   a rooms available for patients' activities?

   b equipment (such as games, easels, wool)?

   c residents using equipment?

13. Isolation room

    a at least one bed and bathroom available for patients with contagious illness?

14. Toilet facilities

    a convenient to bedrooms?

    b easy for a wheelchair patient to use?

    c washbasin?

    d nurse-call bell?

    e handrails on or near toilets?

    f baths and showers with non-slip surfaces?

15. Grounds

    a residents can get fresh air?

    b ramps to help disabled?

SERVICES

16. Medical

    a doctor available in emergency?

    b personal doctor allowed?

    c regular medical attention assured?

    d thorough physical immediately before or upon admission?

    e medical records and plan of care kept?

    f patient involved in developing plans for treatment?

    g other medical services (dentists, opticians, physiotherapists and so on) available regularly?

17. Hospital

    a arrangements with nearby hospital for transfer if necessary?

18. Nursing services

    a registered nurse responsible for nursing staff in a registered nursing home?

    b licensed practical nurse on duty day and night in a registered nursing home?

c trained nurses' aides and orderlies on duty in homes providing some nursing care?

19. Rehabilitation

a specialists in various therapies available when needed?

20. Activities

a individual patient preferences observed?

b group and individual activities?

c residents encouraged but not forced to participate?

d outside trips for those who can go?

e volunteers from the community work with patients?

21. Religious observance

a arrangements made for patients to worship as desired?

b religious observances a matter of choice?

22. Social Services

a social worker available to help residents and families?

23. Food

a planned menus for patients on special diets?

b variety from meal to meal?

c meals served at normal times?

d plenty of time for each meal?

e snacks?

f food delivered to patients' rooms when necessary?

g help with eating given if needed?

ATTITUDES AND ATMOSPHERE

24. General atmosphere friendly and supportive?

25. Residents retain human rights?

a may participate in planning treatment?

b medical records kept confidential?

c can veto experimental research?

d have freedom and privacy to attend to personal needs?

e married couples may share a room?

f all have opportunities to socialize?

g may manage own finances if capable?

h may decorate their own bedrooms?

i may wear their own clothes?

j may communicate with anyone without censorship?

k are not transferred or discharged arbitrarily?

26. Administrators and staff available to discuss problems?

a patients and relatives discuss complaints without fear of reprisal?

b staff respond to calls quickly and courteously?

27. Residents appear alert unless very ill?

28. Residents who are out of bed are wearing day clothes?

29. Visiting hours accommodate residents and relatives?

30. Civil rights regulations observed?

31. Visitors and volunteers pleased with home?

Appendix B

Other Dementias and Related Disorders

Reversible and treatable conditions and disorders producing symptoms similar to the dementia associated with Alzheimer's were discussed in Chapter Two. This Appendix reviews other disorders that may also be considered irreversible dementias or may produce symptoms of dementia at certain stages.[1] Many of the symptoms associated with these disorders are similar to those of Alzheimer's, but others are more specific to the particular disease process. Carer concerns are often very similar, though specific medications used for treatment may differ.

1. Vascular dementia

Vascular dementia is the second most common cause of chronic irreversible dementia in older adults. The older name for one primary type of vascular dementia is *multi-infarct dementia*. Its cause is often multiple strokes or infarcts (necrotic areas) in the brain that occur in blood vessels feeding brain cells, preventing adequate blood flow to areas of the brain; when brain cells are not fed enough oxygen and nutrients because blood flow is cut off, they die. (This process is similar to what happens when someone has a heart attack and blood flow to cells in cardiac tissue is compromised.) There can also be a vascular dementia caused by one single major stroke (*single infarct dementia* or *post-stroke dementia*) versus a series of small strokes. Another name for a stroke is a cerebrovascular accident (CVA). Vascular dementia can also be a corollary to diabetes, past history of heart attacks or other cardiac abnormalities, and hypertension.

Symptoms associated with vascular dementia may seem to appear suddenly, though multiple-stroke or mini-stroke activity has been occurring over a period of time without any obvious symptoms. When symptoms *do* occur there may be periods of confusion similar to symptoms seen in stage one Alzheimer's disease, followed by periods called plateaus when there seems to be no perceptible change in memory or behaviour; this process differs from the slow, steady, global decline associated with Alzheimer's. Persons with vascular dementia may exhibit specific local or focal neurological impairment related to specific areas of brain involvement; for example, slurred speech or muscle weakness in an arm and/or leg. People who have had right-sided strokes often experience cognitive difficulties that vary in degree depending on the location and severity of the stroke. Symptoms include: poor reasoning skills; difficulty with problem solving; difficulty with learning new things; and impairment of recent memory. To complicate diagnosis, Alzheimer's disease and vascular dementia can coexist, and frequently do, in what is called a 'mixed-dementia' that may account for 20 per cent or more of all existing chronic dementias.

Differentiating Alzheimer's from vascular dementia through various neuro-imaging techniques is of great importance; even small strokes can be visualized and lesions in brain tissue will show up on MRI scans. Though vascular dementia is not considered reversible, further stroke activity and associated dementia may be preventable or the risk decreased as many of the risk factors for vascular dementia are known and may be controlled or modified (for example, hypertension, high blood glucose, smoking, high cholesterol, obesity). Surgical, dietary and pharmacological interventions may be indicated as well as other lifestyle changes.

Binswanger's disease, also known as leukoariosis or subcortical leukoencephalopathy, is a rare type of vascular dementia associated with persistent, severe and sustained hypertension. Risk factors also include diabetes, cardiovascular disease and recurrent hypotension. Advanced arteriosclerosis in the medullary arteries occurs with pathologic changes in the frontal subcortical white matter of the brain.

Symptoms of Binswanger's disease include difficulty with

swallowing (dysphagia) and difficulty with thinking, learning and articulating words (dysarthria). Difficulty with walking, frequent falls and urinary incontinence may occur as well. Binswanger's is also plateau-like in progression. Control of associated risk factors may help to slow or halt disease progression. Neuro-imaging techniques are used to diagnose Binswanger's.

A less severe form of small blood vessel disease is called *subcortical vascular dementia*. This is also characterized by walking difficulty and is more gradual in progression.

2. Dementia with Lewy bodies

Dementia with Lewy bodies or DLB (also called *Lewy body dementia*) was first identified in 1983; specific guidelines for diagnosis were formulated in 1996. Lewy bodies are normally found in the brain cells of people with Parkinson's disease in two primary areas, but in DLB these bodies are scattered throughout the brain. The bodies are caused by abnormal protein deposits called alpha-synuclein; they were discovered and described in 1912 by Frederic H. Lewy, a German neurologist and a colleague of Alois Alzheimer. People may have DLB alone or in combination with Alzheimer's disease. DLB is believed to account for approximately 10 to 15 per cent of all dementias in people and generally occurs over the age of sixty-five.

Defining characteristics of DLB include visual hallucinations and Parkinsonism-type symptoms such as muscle rigidity, tremors, a shuffling gait and very slow movement. Onset is more sudden than the more gradually progressing Alzheimer's dementia. There may also be an associated sleep disorder that can result in nightmares, accompanied by periods of drowsiness and lethargy during the day. Research indicates that in about 50 per cent of DLB cases, rapid eye movement (REM) sleep is adversely affected. Normally during REM sleep, people dream but do not 'act out' their dream experiences due to a type of muscle paralysis. If REM sleep is affected by DLB, people can become violent; they may injure themselves or others as they physically act out their dreams. In the daytime, falls may be frequent due to poor balance and fainting spells. Depression is also common.

Symptoms can vary or fluctuate at different times of the day, unlike Alzheimer's symptoms, which tend to remain more constant. The dementia associated with DLB occurs in the early stages of the disease, unlike any dementia associated with Parkinson's. People with DLB may also experience symptoms similar to Alzheimer's dementia, including difficulty with communication and spatial disorientation in addition to memory loss.

There is also a lack of acetylcholine in the brains of people with DLB (similar to Alzheimer's) as well as a deficit of dopamine (similar to Parkinson's). Cholinesterase-inhibitor medications are one treatment that shows promise for the treatment of DLB and they have been used in clinical trials. Neuroleptic (antipsychotic) medications that have a tranquillizing effect and are used to treat psychotic behaviours are not recommended as they block dopamine receptors in the brain and can have adverse effects; for example, muscle rigidity, immobility and even sudden death. Examples of some of the primary neuroleptics are haloperidol (Haldol, Serenace), olanzapine (Zyprexa) and risperidone (Risperdal). In 2004 the Committee on the Safety of Medicines issued a warning that olanzapine and risperidone should not be given to people with dementia. There have been concerns, however, that neuroleptic medications have been prescribed to people with Alzheimer's for behaviours such as agitation and hallucinations even though these medications are only licensed for people with schizophrenia. Medications used to treat Parkinson's disease may be prescribed, although they may also increase confusion and hallucinations. Physiotherapy may help with issues of balance and mobility.

3. Prion-related dementia

Prions are infectious forms of protein that can attack the central nervous system and then invade the brain, causing degeneration of neurons and a build-up of amyloid. Cells that have died take on a sponge-like appearance and the result is a spongiform encephalopathy. While rare, the media has focused on this type of dementia, and carers and the general public often have questions about it and may erroneously equate it with Alzheimer's disease.

Creutzfeldt-Jakob disease (CJD) is a rare form of prion dementia that usually occurs after the age of sixty. Although early symptoms are similar to Alzheimer's, including memory impairment, mood changes and slow or slurred speech, CJD has a very rapid progression. Symptoms may also include shakiness and sudden jerking movements (myoclonus), unsteady gait, an exaggerated startle reflex and epileptic seizures. Total care in the home or nursing home will eventually be needed. Death generally occurs within about six months to a year, and is often associated with pneumonia.

CJD can be diagnosed by brain autopsy following death due to unique pathologic changes in brain tissue; while the sufferer is living, there may be abnormal EEG readings. A spinal tap (lumbar puncture) may also indicate the presence of a substance in cerebrospinal fluid known as '14-3-3 protein'. There is currently no effective treatment for this disease, though some medications may alleviate some of the parkinsonism-type symptoms.

One variant of CJD is bovine spongiform encephalopathy (BSE) or 'mad cow disease', which has been a concern in some parts of the UK and other countries. The concern is related to meat that has been marketed from prion-infected cattle, which may then infect people who eat it. Brains and spinal cords of cattle are now being removed prior to processing beef for human consumption. This infectious disease may account for 5 to 10 per cent of cases of human CJD and can affect people of all age groups.

4. Neurotransmitter abnormalities

Parkinson's disease is caused by the absence of dopamine, a neurotransmitter that controls muscle activity. People with Parkinson's may often experience dementia in the later stages of this illness. In the early stages of Parkinson's, slowed or delayed thinking processes may be evident but, unlike Alzheimer's, a person with Parkinson's, given time, will usually be able to remember and reason even though speech may be slower than normal. These two diseases are often confused in both early and late stages.

To confuse matters more, persons with Parkinson's may actually

develop Alzheimer's, and persons with Alzheimer's may exhib
symptoms more typically characteristic of Parkinson's – for exampl
lack of facial expression, increased muscle tone and joint stiffnes
slow movement (bradykinesia), difficulty with walking (shufflin
or initiating movement, stooped posture and sometimes comple
immobility. One feature unique to Parkinson's disease and usual
absent in Alzheimer's is tremors or mild to severe shaking of th
hands and head.

Medication can help alleviate symptoms associated wit
Parkinson's, specifically the medication levodopa or L-dop
Antidepressants are also often ordered to combat depression, whic
is frequently associated with the disease.

5. Hereditary dementias

Huntington's disease or *Huntington's chorea* is a hereditar
disorder involving early stage cognitive changes, short-ter
memory impairment and involuntary movements (chorea) of th
face and upper extremities. Depression, hallucinations and parano
may also occur early in the disease and progression may be a slo
deterioration. People with Huntington's generally continue
recognize loved ones.

A genetic marker identified on chromosome 4 has been linke
to the Huntington's gene. Pathologic changes in the brain inclu
marked atrophy, extensive nerve cell loss and a decrease in whi
matter. Age of onset is generally between thirty and forty-five yea
or later.

Various medications may help control abnormal musc
movements, though they often lead to rigidity as a side effe
Antidepressants are often used to combat depression, though the
is no specific treatment for the associated dementia.

6. Fronto-temporal dementias

There are a number of *fronto-temporal dementias* that may va
with respect to the specific changes that occur in the frontal a
anterior temporal lobes of the brain. Common symptoms inclu

early and marked personality changes such as apathy and lack of empathy and concern for other people, irritability, compulsive or ritualistic behaviours, cravings for specific foods (especially sweets), loss of inhibitions and inappropriate sexual behaviour, and lack of attention to dressing and grooming. Speech is often affected and the person may have difficulty finding the right words to say or forming words at all, or might use too many words. Generally there is no initial memory loss and memory and cognition are not as dramatically affected in later stages, unlike Alzheimer's. Fronto-temporal dementias may be diagnosed by neuro-imaging techniques such as MRIs and PET scans; atrophy (shrinkage) of the frontal and temporal lobes may be present and certain areas in the brain may indicate low metabolism. A detailed history of symptoms and symptom progression obtained from friends and family members may help differentiate fronto-temporal dementia from other types of dementia. Fronto-temporal dementia accounts for about 10 per cent of all dementias; it can develop between the ages of thirty-five and seventy-five. Non-pharmacological strategies similar to those used for people with Alzheimer's are usually the most helpful interventions. Many medications used to treat other types of dementia may worsen symptoms and increase aggressive behaviour.

Primary progressive aphasis is a subtype of fronto-temporal dementia. There is a loss of language ability initially but no early signs of memory loss, unlike Alzheimer's. It may be confused with depression.

Fronto-temporal dementia with Parkinsonism may also occur and is related to a mutation in a gene linked to chromosome 17. Symptoms may be similar to Parkinson's, although there are generally no tremors at rest.

Pick's disease (PKD) is a rarer fronto-temporal lobar dementia that often manifests itself in disturbances of mood and a progressive inability to speak (aphasia), which may render a person totally mute. Disinhibitions of a sexual nature, inappropriate social behaviours and loss of social awareness are more indicative of Pick's than of traditional Alzheimer's dementia; memory loss is not as profound as in Alzheimer's disease. Behavioural disturbances may occur later in the disease and may include hyperorality (overeating) and visual agnosia (inability to interpret visual images). PKD initially affects people in their fifties and sixties.

Like Alzheimer's, Pick's disease can best be diagnosed by brain autopsy. Autopsy can reveal plaques and tangles, loss of brain tissue, and 'Pick bodies' in the cerebral cortex, basal ganglia and some brainstem structures. On a CAT scan, severe atrophy may be present, especially in the temporal and frontal areas of the brain.

There is no cure for fronto-temporal dementias but some medications are used for symptom management.

7. Motor neuron abnormalities

Amyotrophic lateral sclerosis (ALS), a motor neuron abnormality (also called 'Lou Gehrig's disease' after the famous US baseball player who developed it), is characterized by progressive muscle wasting and weakness, involuntary contractions of the face and tongue, atrophy and difficulty speaking, and spasticity. ALS may be due to an excess of the chemical glutamate, which is responsible for relaying messages between motor neurons. Too much glutamate destroys nerve cells in the brain and spinal column.

Recent research indicates that some people with ALS will experience problems with memory and decision-making and may develop additional symptoms of dementia as the disease progresses. ALS is commonly seen in people in their late thirties and forties.

8. White matter abnormalities

Multiple sclerosis (MS) is a progressive, degenerative disease affecting the myelin sheath and conduction pathway involvement of the central nervous system. White fibre tracts connecting white matter and neurons in the brain and spinal column are usually affected. Causative explanations include viral, immunologic and genetic factors. CT scanning may show increased density in the white matter and MS plaques. MRI and PET scanning may also be used to diagnose.

As MS progresses, memory loss, impaired judgement, and an inability to problem solve and perform calculations may occur. Earlier symptoms include generalized muscle weakness, fatigue, tremors when performing activities, numbness and tingling sensations, visual disturbances, mood swings, dizziness and ringing in the ears, and disturbances with bowel and bladder function.

Because symptoms are often vague and can mimic other diseases, MS often goes undiagnosed and cognitive symptoms can easily be misinterpreted as Alzheimer's disease. Symptoms of MS typically occur in the twenty to forty-year-old age range.

9. Disorders related to alcohol excess and vitamin deficiency

Wernicke-Korsakoff syndrome is a condition that can develop which results in a type of irreversible dementia with memory loss. It is generally related to chronic alcoholism that results in a thiamine (Vitamin B1) deficiency. Thiamine is needed by the brain cells to convert sugar into energy. The initial acute stage is called *Wernicke encephalopathy*; the chronic stage that follows is called *Korsakoff psychosis*.

Symptoms are confusion, confabulation (filling in memory gaps with inappropriate words or fabricated ideas) and lack of coordination related to muscle weakness. Early intervention with high doses of thiamine and abstinence from alcohol may reverse some of the brain damage, but generally not all.

Appendix C

Research and Medications

Research and the development of new experimental drugs is ongoing and ever-changing. Clinical drug trials are being conducted in the UK, the US and a number of other countries in Europe. There is also a drug regulatory system in Europe and many steps must be taken before marketing approval is given in European countries. For fact sheets and information on these experimental drug studies, contact the Alzheimer's Society or view their website (see Appendix D). The following is a brief summary of some of the latest and most significant developments in Alzheimer's research.

1. Amyloid protein research and medications

Researchers have long studied the beta-amyloid protein, a sticky substance that accumulates in the brains of persons with Alzheimer's disease and forms plaques, one primary characteristic of Alzheimer's. Recent research suggests that this protein also produces free radicals, or molecules with odd numbers of electrons, which in turn are known to cause cell damage or cell death. Recently, British and US researchers introduced an adapted piece of the enzyme ABAD into the nerve cells of mice and observed that brain cells injected with ABAD were not damaged by beta-amyloid in the same way as other brain cells. It is possible a similar mechanism might prevent beta-amyloid forming in the human brain.

Proteins called *secretases* are known to act on amyloid precursor proteins in the brain and promote the production of beta-amyloid. Researchers are developing drugs they hope will block or inhibit the production of beta-amyloid. One drug undergoing human trials is R-flurbiprofen (Flurizan) produced by Myriad Phamaceuticals. Antiaggregate medications may also block beta-amyloid production. NC-758 Alzhemed drug trials are also underway.

Earlier research has shown that some antioxidants serve to protect cells from naturally occurring free-radical damage. Clinical trials have included the medication selegiline (Deprenyl), which is believed to block free-radical damage and improve memory. Selegiline has antioxidant properties and is now a fully licensed medication in the UK. Vitamin E may also serve to neutralize the toxic effects of free radicals. People with diets higher in vitamin E appear to have a lower risk of developing Alzheimer's. Foods high in vitamin E include leafy darker green vegetables, vegetable oils, nuts (almonds, hazelnuts, sunflower seeds), peanut butter, fortified cereals, wheat germ (that can be sprinkled on cereal), chicken, turkey and liver, and seafoods such as salmon, scallops and shrimp. Carers should not give their loved ones excess doses of over-the-counter vitamin E. Excess doses of any vitamin are highly toxic, and excess vitamin E supplementation may increase risks for stroke (cardiovascular accidents).

There have also been some vaccine studies conducted based on the theory that a vaccine could mobilize the immune system to produce antibodies that would attack beta-amyloid and prevent or reverse the process of plaque formation. The vaccines would be used to treat people with Alzheimer's rather than be given to prevent it from occurring. Studies have shown inconclusive results. Trials were discontinued in 2002 when some study participants died, but research continues to develop vaccines that are less toxic, as some vaccinated subjects did appear to have a slower progression of the disease. Many experts believe this research is one of the most promising lines of enquiry.

2. The genetic question

In 1987 researchers discovered evidence for a gene or genes on chromosome 21 related to Alzheimer's disease specifically in some families with early-onset familial Alzheimer's disease (FAD). FAD occurs in about 1 to 10 per cent of all persons with Alzheimer's disease and has been known to occur in persons in their thirties. Chromosome 21 is the same chromosome associated with the occurrence of Down's syndrome; abnormalities in the brain that occur in persons with Down's syndrome by the age of forty are similar to those occurring in people with Alzheimer's, including the characteristic plaques and tangles. Also in 1987, the gene that contains the code for the amyloid precursor protein (APP) was found on chromosome 21. APP is related to beta-amyloid protein and senile plaque formation.

In 1992 the APP gene on chromosome 14 was found to contain a mutation(s) associated with some early-onset familial Alzheimer's disease cases that affected persons in their forties.

In 1993 chromosome 19 was found to have a genetic mutation that was more than three times as common in persons with both late-onset FAD and sporadic AD (no 'known' relatives had Alzheimer's disease) than in persons without Alzheimer's disease. This gene is called apolipoprotein E (ApoE). ApoE appears to be the first biological risk factor for late-onset Alzheimer's (other than age itself). The study of the ApoE gene is one of the most promising avenues of research. In the future there may be ways to reduce a person's risk of developing Alzheimer's – for example, by manipulating metabolism to postpone Alzheimer's – according to Duke University researchers in the US.

There are several types of the ApoE gene: ApoE2, ApoE3 and ApoE4. A higher risk for developing Alzheimer's is associated with ApoE4. ApoE3 appears to account for the development of Alzheimer's in the very old (over the age of eighty). People with the ApoE2 gene appear to be at lowest risk. The ApoE gene is also a risk factor for vascular dementia.

A collaboration of experts in the UK led by researchers at Cardiff University is currently conducting a study of the entire human genome in the hope of identifying genes that predispose people to Alzheimer's or protect people from developing Alzheimer's. This study is funded by the Welcome Trust, the UK's largest charity. DNA samples will be taken from 14,000 people (6,000 with late-onset Alzheimer's and 8,000 healthy control subjects) from the UK and

US; common genetic variations that increase the risk for Alzheimer's will be explored. Genes that affect cholesterol levels, for example, are believed to increase the risk of Alzheimer's disease.

The Alzheimer's Society UK has a helpful fact sheet entitled 'Genetics and dementia'. This includes useful information that gives the pros and cons of genetic testing. A printable version of the fact sheet is available on their main website (www.alzheimers.org.uk).

3. Environmental factors

The primary risk factor for Alzheimer's disease is age. Statistics from the Alzheimer's Society indicate that one in fifty people between the ages of sixty-five and seventy have some form of dementia; one in five have some form of dementia after the age of eighty. Women are slightly more at risk of Alzheimer's disease than men; men are more likely to develop vascular dementia. Specific medical conditions also appear to be risk factors for the development of vascular dementia – for example, hypertension, high blood cholesterol, and a history of stroke, diabetes or heart abnormalities.

Researchers believe some factor(s) in the environment may play a part in the development of Alzheimer's disease. The study of various metals in the environment such as aluminium, mercury, copper and zinc is ongoing. To date the research has yielded mixed results.

Chelation therapy is sometimes advertised in popular self-help magazines as a means of ridding the body of excess aluminium or zinc. But the side effects, including hypotension, vomiting, anaemia, irregular heartbeat, congestive heart failure and kidney failure, far outweigh the proposed benefits. Carers should seek advice from the Alzheimer's Society or a reputable medical centre before subjecting their loved one to any alternative treatment.

Another environmental area of exploration is related to electromagnetic fields (EMFs) from power lines and other electrical equipment. A study reported in the *American Journal of Epidemiology* in September 1995 found increased likelihood of dementia in persons exposed to frequent and high levels of EMFs; this research needs to be replicated before conclusions can be reached about possible links between Alzheimer's and EMFs.

Long-term exposure to pesticides is also considered to be a possible risk factor for dementia and is under investigation. Smoking also increases the risk for dementia due to its effect on the respiratory and cardiovascular system. This includes blood vessels in the brain.

4. Acetylcholine research and related medications

Drugs that are acetylcholinesterase inhibitors have been approved for use in the US, the UK, Australia and some other countries. These medications reduce the breakdown of the neurotransmitter acetylcholine at the synaptic gap by inhibiting production of acetylcholinesterase; this in turn makes more acetylcholine available to enhance communication between cells (see also Chapter Four).

A number of anticholinesterase drugs (also called acetylcholinesterase inhibitors) have been tested in clinical trials. The experimental medication tacrine (Cognex) was first tested in 1986. It was approved by the US Food and Drug Administration as the first drug released for the treatment of mild to moderate Alzheimer's. It is rarely if ever prescribed today due to associated side effects, for example, liver damage.

Donepezil hydrochloride (Aricept), produced by Eisai and co-marketed with Pfizer, was the first drug licensed specifically for mild to moderate Alzheimer's in the UK, in 1997. Rivastigmine (Exelon), produced by Novartis Pharmaceuticals, was the second drug licensed in the UK for Alzheimer's. The Alzheimer's Society notes it can temporarily slow down the progression of symptoms in people with mild to moderate dementia. This medication is available in pill form and also as a once-daily trans-dermal patch.

Galantamine (Reminyl) is an acetylcholinesterase inhibitor recommended for mild to moderately severe Alzheimer's dementia. Galantamine appears to stimulate nicotinic receptors in the brain; researchers believe this stimulation helps to replace the action of the acetylcholine normally destroyed by Alzheimer's. It is available in capsule form.

None of the cholinesterase inhibitors are cures for Alzheimer's but they have had positive effects on symptoms in the mild to moderate stages – for example, improved memory, language and decision-making ability, and improved ability to carry out activities of daily living, such as dressing and toileting. On average, these medications may delay or slow the worsening of symptoms for six to twelve months for about 50 per cent of the people who take them, according to the US Alzheimer's Association. Side effects are minimized by starting these medications at a low dose and gradually increasing the dosage.

Fact sheets are available through the Alzheimer's Society and through the drug manufacturers for the primary approved medications. This includes possible side effects. The most common ones are nausea, vomiting, appetite loss and more frequent bowel movements.

NMDA receptors (ionotropic receptors for glutamate are also involved in transmitting nerve signals for learning and remembering. Some drugs that are being researched belong to a category called NMDA-receptor antagonists. Memantine (marketed as Namenda in the US and Ebixa in the UK) was the first medication approved in the US to treat moderate to severe dementia as a result of its effectiveness in clinical trials compared with a placebo; subjects in one large-scale study taking memantine showed significantly less cognitive deterioration and a greater ability to perform activities of daily living than those taking a placebo. Memantine is also supported by experts in the UK for similar treatment. Randomized double-blind clinical trials have shown improvement in cognitive and behavioural symptoms including ability to perform activities of daily living in people with moderate to severe Alzheimer's. Memantine helps to facilitate the transmission of nerve signals by regulating the activity of glutamate, a chemical that triggers the NMDA receptors to allow controlled amounts of calcium into nerve cells. Calcium is essential for information storage. Too much calcium, however, can cause cellular death. It is believed that memantine may partially block NMDA receptors and protect against excess glutamate secretion. Side effects include headaches, confusion, dizziness, hallucinations and constipation; all can generally be alleviated with adjusted doses. Memantine was created by Merz Pharmaceuticals and was approved for use in Europe in 2002; it may also be given in combination with another medication such as donepezil.

5. Mitochondria research and supplements

Mitochondria are slender microscopic filaments or organelles (little organs) in body cells. They are considered to be the source of energy for cells and are involved in protein synthesis and lipid or fat metabolism. Acetyl-L-carnitine hydrochloride naturally occurs in human cells (especially heart, muscle and brain cells) and effects the proper functioning of mitochondria. Mitochondrial decay appears to be related to ageing. The drug Alcar (acetyl-L-carnitine) is currently being tested on an experimental basis at a number of sites in the US. In one relatively small-sample study, subjects with probable Alzheimer's who received acetyl-L-carnitine showed significantly less deterioration in their mini-mental status examinations and Alzheimer's Disease Assessment Scale test scores than those who received a placebo. Alcar is sold over the counter as an anti-ageing supplement; carers should check with their GP about dosage if they are considering it as a treatment option.

6. Other alternative medications

Ginkgo biloba is a popular over-the-counter supplement stocked by pharmacies and health food shops; primary claims for it are improvement of memory and circulation. Ginkgo biloba extract is derived from dried leaves of the ginkgo (maidenhair) tree that is native to China. There have been a number of studies conducted on Ginkgo related to improving cognition and there is currently a large randomized trial underway in the US with 3,000 people enrolled called the Gingko Evaluation of Memory (GEM) study; effects of Ginkgo on memory, thinking and personality will be examined. Study results are expected by 2008. The study is sponsored by the National Center for Complimentary and Alternative Medicine, the National Heart, Lung and Blood Institute and the National Institute on Ageing; all agencies are affiliated with the National Institutes of Health.

Ginkgo has been studied and more extensively prescribed for treatment of circulatory conditions and dementia by doctors in Europe than in the US. As with any alternative medication, it is important to discuss it with your doctor. If your loved one is on anticoagulant therapy (for example, warfarin or aspirin) or there are any associated problems with blood clotting, Ginkgo may be contraindicated.

The Alzheimer's Society has a useful information sheet on complementary and alternative medicine and dementia, which contains the most recent information about related research. This includes other types of therapy such as aromatherapy, massage and music therapy.

Appendix D

Useful Organizations and Resources

(See primary UK websites for information about similar organizations in Scotland, Ireland and Wales)

Action on Elder Abuse
Astral House
1268 London Road
Norbury
London SW16 4ER
Tel: 020 8765 7000
Fax: 020 8679 4074
Email: enquiries@elderabuse.org.uk
UK helpline: 0808 808 8141

Age Concern Cymru (Wales)
Ty John Pathy
13/14 Neptune Court
Vanguard Way
Cardiff CF24 5PJ
Tel: 029 2043 1555
Fax: 029 2047 1418
Email: enquiries@accymru.org.uk
http://www.accymru.org.uk

Age Concern England
Astral House
1268 London Road
Norbury
London SW16 4ER
Tel: 020 8765 7200
Free information helpline: 0800 00 99 66
Email: ace@ace.org.uk
http://www.ageconcern.org.uk

Age Concern Northern Ireland
3 Lower Crescent
Belfast BT7 1NR
Tel: +44(0)28 9024 5729
Fax: +44(0)28 9023 5479
Email: info@ageconcernni.org
http://www.ageconcernni.org

Age Concern Scotland
Causewayside House
160 Causewayside
Edinburgh EH9 1PR
Tel: 0845 833 0200
Fax: 0845 833 0759
Freephone: 0800 00 99 66 (7am–7pm, 7 days a week)
Email: enquiries@acsot.org.uk
http://www.ageconcernscotland.org.uk

Alzheimer Scotland
22 Drumsheugh Gardens
Edinburgh EH3 7RN
Tel: 0131 243 1453
Fax: 0131 243 1450
Email: alzheimer@alzscot.org
http://www.alzscot.org/

Alzheimer's Society (UK)
Gordon House
10 Greencoat Place
London SWIP 1PH
Tel: 020 7306 0606
Fax: 020 7306 0808
Email: enquiries@alzheimers.org.uk
http://www.alzheimers.org.uk/

The Alzheimer Society of Ireland
National Office (see website for regional offices)
Alzheimer House
43 Northumberland Avenue
Dun Laoghaire, Co Dublin
Tel: (01) 284 6616
National helpline: (01) 800 341 341
Fax: (01) 284 6030
Email: info@alzheimer.ie
http://www.alzheimer.ie/

Association of Community Health Partnerships
Jim Laing, Secretary
70 Turnberry Gardens
Westerwood
Cumbernauld
Glasgow G68 0AZ
Tel/Fax: 01236 457 853
Email: laing.jim@btinternet.com
http://www.achp.scot.nhs.uk/

At Dementia (Assistive Technologies)
Trent Dementia Services Development Centre
9 Newarke Street
Leicester LE1 5SN
Tel: 0116 257 5017
Fax: 0116 254 3983
Email: info@trentdsdc.org.uk
http://www.atdementia.org.uk

Attendance Allowance Unit, DSS
Warbreck House
Warbreck Hill
Blackpool
Lancashire FY2 0YE
Helpline: 08457 123 456
Textphone: 08457 224 433
Email: DCPU.Customer-Services@dwp.gsi.gov.uk
http://www.dwp.gov.uk/lifeevent/benefits/dcs/contact_dcs.asp
http://www.direct.gov.uk/en/Dl1/Directories/DG_10011169

British Red Cross
UK Office
44 Moorfields
London EC2Y 9AL
Tel: 0870 170 7000
Fax: 020 7562 2000
http://www.redcross.org.uk

Carers UK
20–25 Glasshouse Yard
London EC1A 4JT
Tel: 020 7490 8818
Fax: 020 7490 8824
Email: info@carersuk.org
http://www.carersuk.org/Contactus (for contacts in Ireland, Scotland & Wales)

Carer's Allowance Unit
Department of Work and Pensions
Palatine House
Lancaster Road
Preston
Lancashire PR1 1HB
Tel: 01253 856 123
http://www.dwp.gov.uk

Citizens advice information
http://www.citizensadvice.org.uk
http://www.adviceguide.org.uk/

Commission for Social Care Inspection
33 Greycoat Street
London SW1P 2QF
Tel: 020 7979 2000
Fax: 020 7979 2111
Helpline number: 0845 015 0120
Helpline number (Newcastle): 0191 233 3323
Email: enquiries@csci.gsi.gov.uk
http://www.csci.org.uk/

Counsel and Care for Older People and their Carers
Twyman House
16 Bonny Street
London NW1 9PG
Advice line telephone enquiries: 0845 300 7585 (Local Call Rate)
General telephone enquiries: 020 7241 8555
Email: advice@counselandcare.org.uk
http://www.counselandcare.org.uk/contact-us/

Crossroads Association (Caring for Carers)
10 Regent Place
Rugby
Warwickshire CV21 2PN
Tel: 0845 450 0350
Fax: 0845 450 6556
http://www.crossroads.org.uk/

Dementia Voice
Hillside Court
Batten Road
Bristol BS5 8NL
Tel: 0870 192 4747
Fax: 0870 192 4748
Email: kim.warren@housing21.co.uk
http://www.dementia-voice.org.uk

**Dial UK (The National Association of
Disablement Information and Advice Lines)**
Park Lodge
St Catherine's Hospital
Tickhill Road
Doncaster
South Yorkshire DN4 8QN
Tel: 01302 310 123
Fax: 01302 310 404
Textphone: 01302 310 123 (please use voice announcer)
Email: informationenquiries@dialuk.org.uk
http://www.dialuk.info/

Disability Alliance
Universal House
88–94 Wentworth Street
London E1 7SA
Tel: 020 7247 8776
http://www.disabilityalliance.org/

Disability Living Allowance Unit
Warbreck House
Warbreck Hill
Blackpool
Lancashire FY2 0YE
Helpline: 08457 123 456
Textphone: 08457 224 433
Email: DCPU.Customer-Services@dwp.gsi.gov.uk
http://www.dwp.gov.uk/lifeevent/benefits/dcs/contact_dcs.asp
http://www.direct.gov.uk/en/Dl1/Directories/DG_10011169

Disabled Living Foundation
380–384 Harrow Road
London W9 2HU
Helpline: 0845 130 9177
Textphone: 020 7432 8009
Email: advice@dlf.org.uk
General email: info@dlf.org.uk
http://www.dlf.org.uk/about/contact.html

Driver and Vehicle Licensing Agency (DVLA)
Tel: 0870 240 0009
Email: drivers.dvla@gtnet.gov.uk
http://www.dvla.gov.uk/medical/medical_advisory_information.aspx

Elderly Accommodation Counsel (EAC)
3rd Floor, 89 Albert Embankment
London SE1 7TP
Tel: 020 7820 1343
Fax: 020 7820 3970
http://www.housingcare.org
http://www.eac.org.uk

ERoSH
The Essential Role of Sheltered Housing
National Housing Consortium
PO Box 2616
Chippenham
Wiltshire SN15 1WZ
Tel/Fax: 01249 654 249
Email: info@shelteredhousing.org
http://www.shelteredhousing.org/

For Dementia
6 Camden High Street
London NW1 0JH
Tel: 020 7874 7210
Fax: 020 7874 7219
http://www.fordementia.org.uk
http://www.patient.co.uk/showdoc/26738972/

Help The Aged
207–221 Pentonville Road
London N1 9UZ
Tel: 020 7278 1114
Email: info@helptheaged.org.uk
http://www.helptheaged.org.uk/en-gb/WhatWeDo/AboutUs/ContactUs/

Holiday Care Service
Tourism for All
The Hawkins Suite
Enham Place
Enham Alamein
Andover SP11 6JS
Tel: 0845 124 9971
Minicom: 0845 124 9976
Fax: 0845 124 9972
Email: info@tourismforall.org.uk
http://www.holidaycare.org.uk/

Invalid Care Allowance Unit, DSS
Palatine House
Lancaster Road
Preston
Lancashire PR1 1HB
Tel: 01772 899508
http://www.dss.gov.uk/lifeevent/benefits/carers_allowance.asp

Law Centres Federation
293–299 Kentish Town Road
London NW5 2TJ
Tel: 020 7428 4400
Fax: 020 7428 4401
Email: info@lawcentres.org.uk
http://www.lawcentres.org.uk/

MIND (National Association for Mental Health)
Granta House
15–19 Broadway
London E15 4BQT
Tel: 020 8519 2122
Email: contact@mind.org.uk
http://www.mind.org.uk/

National Association of Citizens Advice Bureau
Myddelton House
115–23 Pentonville Road
London N1 9LZ
http://www.adviceguide.org.uk/

Office of the Public Guardian
Tel: 0845 330 2900
http://www.publicguardian.gov.uk/

Parish Nursing Ministries UK
Revd Helen Wordsworth
3 Barnwell Close
Dunchurch
Nr Rugby
Warwickshire CV22 6QH
Tel: 01788 817292
http://www.parishnursing.co.uk/

The Princess Royal Trust for Carers
London Office
142 Minories
London EC3N 1LB
Tel: 020 7480 7788
Fax: 020 7481 4729
For publications and PR email: Info (info@carers.org)
For all other enquiries email: Help Desk (help@carers.org)
http://www.carers.org/

The Public Trust Office (for legal information)
Protection Division
Stewart House
24 Kingsway
London WC2B 6JX
Tel: 020 7664 7000

Registered Nursing Home Association
15 Highfield Road
Edgbaston
Birmingham B16 8QY
Tel: 0121 454 2511
Email: info@rnha.co.uk
http://www.rnha.co.uk/news/nr010205.htm

Relatives and Residents Association
24 The Ivories
6–18 Northampton Street
London N1 2HY
Tel (Advice Line): 020 7359 8136 (9.30am–4.30pm, Monday–Friday)
Tel (Admin): 020 7359 8148
Fax: 020 7226 6603
http://www.relres.org

St Andrew's Ambulance Association
St Andrew's House
48 Milton Street
Glasgow G4 0HR
Tel: 0141 332 4031
Email: firstaid@staaa.org.uk
http://www.standrewsambulance.org.uk/index.htm
http:www.firstaid.org.uk

St John's Ambulance Brigade
27 St John's Lane
London EC1M 4BU
Tel: 08700 10 49 50
http://www.sja.org.uk/sja/

Scottish Disability Equality Forum
12 Enterprise House
Springkerse Business Park
Stirling FK7 7UF
Tel: 01786 446456
Email: general@sdef.org.uk
http://www.sdef.org.uk/

UK Wandering Network (UKWN)
Dementia inc. Alzheimer's
Email: jan.dewing@btinternet.com
http://www.wanderingnetwork.co.uk

Veterans UK
Service Personnel and Veterans Agency
Norcross
Thornton Cleveleys
Lancashire FY5 3WP
Freephone: 0800 169 22 7
Email: veterans.help@spva.gsi.gov.uk
http://www.veterans-uk.info/faqs/welfare.html7 (UK only)

Wandering in Dementia
WanderGuardian
Tel: 0845 8900200
Lines open Monday to Friday 9am–5pm
Email: eleanor@WanderingInDementia.co.uk
http://www.wanderingindementia.com/index.html

Winslow Press Catalogue
WINSLOW®
Goyt Side Road
Chesterfield
Derbyshire S40 2PH
Tel: 0845 230 2777 (UK) or + 44 1 246 210470
Email: sales@winslow-cat.com
http://www.winslow-press.co.uk/cgi-bin/Winslow.storefront

Youth Access
1–2 Taylor's Yard
67 Alderbrook Road
London SW12 8AD
Tel: 020 8772 9900
Email: admin@youthaccess.org.uk
http://www.youthaccess.org.uk/

Notes

CHAPTER ONE

1. Statistics about Alzheimer's disease and dementia are based on information from the Alzheimer's Society UK. Information can be viewed at: http://www.alzheimers.org.uk/site/ and from Alzheimer's Disease International http://www.alz.co.uk/

See also Knapp, M., Prince, M. et al. (2007) *Dementia UK* (A report to the Alzheimer's Society on the prevalence and economic cost of dementia in the UK produced by King's College London and London School of Economics), Alzheimer's Society: London.

2. *The 36-Hour Day*, by Nancy L. Mace and Peter V. Rabins, is a classic in the field of dementia (New York: Johns Hopkins University Press, Warner Books, 1991. Revised 2001).

CHAPTER TWO

1. M. F Mendez; A. R. Mastri; J. H. Sung; and W. H. Frey (1992) 'Clinically Diagnosed Alzheimer's Disease: Neuropathologic Findings in 650 Cases', *Alzheimer's Disease and Associated Disorders* 6, 35–43. Brain autopsy results on persons previously diagnosed with Alzheimer's disease showed 78 per cent had been correctly diagnosed when living.

2. John Stirling Meyer, Kazuhiro Muramatsu, Karl F. Mortel, Katsuyuki Obara and Toshitaka Shirai (1995) 'Prospective CT Confirms Differences Between Vascular and Alzheimer's Dementia', *Stroke* 26, 735–42.

3. Linda Teri (1994) 'Behavioral Treatment of Depression in Patients with Dementia', *Alzheimer's Disease and Associated Disorders* 8, Suppl. 3 66–74.

4. Two examples of mental state assessment tools are the Mini-Mental State Exam and the Blessed-Roth Dementia Scale (M. E Folstein, S. A. Folstein and P. R. McHugh (1975) 'Mini Mental State: A Practical Method for Grading the Cognitive State of Patients for the Clinician', *Journal of Psychiatric Research* 12, no. 3 189–98; G. Blessed, B. E. Tomlinson and M. Roth (1988) 'Blessed-Roth Dementia Scale', *Psychopharmacology Bulletin* 24, no. 4 705–708.

5. Robert D. Terry, Robert Katzman, Katherine L. Bick and Sangram S. Sisodia, eds. *Alzheimer's Disease* (1999) 2nd edition (Philadelphia: Lippincott, Williams, & Wilkins). A book written for health-care professionals, but also an excellent source of more detailed information for family carers seeking medical references on the diagnostic and treatment aspects of dementia.

CHAPTER THREE

1. Lewis Thomas, *The Medusa and the Snail* (New York: Viking Press, 1979), pp. 169–70.

2. William R. Markesbery and William D. Ehmann, 'Brain Trace Elements in Alzheimer's Disease', in *Alzheimer's Disease*, eds. Terry, Katzman and Bick (New York: Raven Press, 1994), pp. 353–67.

3. For further information about agencies and resources, see Appendix D.

4. The new government website for carers info is:
http://www.direct.gov.uk/en/CaringForSomeone/DG_071391

CHAPTER FOUR

1. Other neurotransmitters under investigation are norepinephrine, serotonin, somatostatin and corticotrophin-releasing factor. All are believed to be deficient in persons with Alzheimer's disease.

2. Alzheimer's disease is staged in a variety of ways in the research literature; no two people progress exactly alike.

CHAPTER FIVE

1. Naomi Feil has developed workshops and resource material on communicating with the old who are confused, focusing on their feelings. She calls her technique 'Validation Therapy'. See Naomi Feil, *The Validation Breakthrough: Simple Techniques for Communicating with People with Alzheimer's-Type Dementia*, 2nd revised edition (Health Professions Press, 2002).

CHAPTER SIX

1. There are a number of books available on communicating with people with dementia. One that has been recommended by professional carers is *Communication and the Care of People with Dementia* by John Killick and Kate Allan (Open University Press, 2001).

CHAPTER SEVEN

1. See http://ods.od.nih.gov/factsheets/vitamind.asp. Ultraviolet (UV) rays from the sun trigger vitamin D synthesis in the skin.

2. A volunteer walker's programme was instituted by Sharon Holmberg (R.N., Ph.D) at St John's Nursing Home in Rochester, New York, providing a supervised hour of walking in the early evening for persons with dementia.

CHAPTER EIGHT

1. See website of the British Nutrition Foundation for more information on various food groups related to age groups (http://www.nutrition.org.uk/).

2. There is a very helpful site from the Heimlich Institute with pictures indicating how to do it on yourself or another person. See http://www. heimlichinstitute.org/page.php?id=34.
This PatientPlus website provides comprehensive, free, up-to-date health information, as provided by GPs to patients during consultations; articles are more technical but provide more in-depth information for carers. See http://www.patient.co.uk/showdoc/40001960/

3. Lore K. Wright, *Alzheimer's Disease and Marriage* (Newbury Park: Sage Publications, 1993), p. 7.

CHAPTER NINE

1. A very useful publication available free to carers called *At the Crossroads: Family Conversations about Alzheimer's Disease, Dementia and Driving* was developed by The Hartford Financial Services Group, Inc. This company conducted research with carers and people with dementia to learn more about how families perceive and manage driving and transportation issues when a loved one has dementia. Some of the information about regulations is specific to the United States but the general family related information would be helpful to carers in any country. Included, for example, are twenty-eight warning signs of driving problems. To access this information with many other useful tips on driving when diagnosed with dementia, see:
http://www.thehartford.com/alzheimers/faq.html

The UK Alzheimer's Society also has a very helpful position statement on driving with a diagnosis of dementia. See http://www.alzheimers.org.uk/site/scripts/documents_info.php?documentID=436

CHAPTER TEN

1. A variety of downloadable brochures, including several for and about teens and children, are available at the following website:
http://www.alz.org/alzheimers_disease_publications_alz_basics.asp

CHAPTER ELEVEN

1. See the Carers UK website for questions and answers about this new ruling, who qualifies as a carer and suggestions for working with employers to meet both personal and company needs.
http://www.carersuk.org/Newsandcampaigns/makeWORKwork/WorkandFamiliesActFAQ

2. This fact sheet includes a very useful list of organizations, and answers carer questions about available resources and costs. It can be downloaded at:
http://www.ageconcern.org.uk/AgeConcern/fs6.asp

3. See http://www.shelteredhousing.org/ for comprehensive information on sheltered housing from ERoSH (The Essential Role of Sheltered Housing).

4. See the Nursing Homes Registry website for a listing of nursing and residential homes in the UK and the services they offer:
http://www.nursinghomes.co.uk/

5. Addresses, phone numbers and websites of agencies discussed in this chapter can be found in Appendix D. Publications titles may change. Many are available on-line through the agencies listed.

CHAPTER TWELVE

1. Granger Westberg, *Good Grief* (Philadelphia: Fortress Press, 1971), p. 20.

2. C. S. Bréitner (1991) 'Clinical Genetics and Genetic Counselling in Alzheimer's Disease', *Annals of Internal Medicine* 115, no. 8: 601–606.

3. See http://www.downs-syndrome.org.uk/DSA_Faqs.aspx. An excellent article on Down's syndrome and Alzheimer's is: Lisa R. Stanton and Rikus H. Coetzee (2004) 'Down's syndrome and dementia' *Advances in Psychiatric Treatment*. Vol. 10, 50–58. This can be viewed on-line at: http://apt.rcpsych.org/cgi/reprint/10/1/50.pdf

4. Karl Menninger, *Whatever Became of Sin?* (New York: Hawthorn Books, 1973), pp. 1–2.

CHAPTER THIRTEEN

1. Anyone who was confused in the nursing home I worked in was diagnosed with chronic organic brain syndrome (COBS); there was little attempt to differentiate various types of dementia.

2. Hugh Silvester, *Arguing with God* (Downers Grove: InterVarsity Press, 1972).

3. C. S. Lewis, *A Grief Observed* (New York: Bantam Books, 1976), pp. 34–35.

4. Christopher Fitzsimons Allison, *Guilt, Anger and God* (New York: Seabury Press, 1972).

5. Quote attributed to Martin Luther in Thomas McCormick and Sharon Fish, *Meditation: A Practical Guide to a Spiritual Discipline* (Downers Grove: InterVarsity Press, 1983), p. 10.

CHAPTER FOURTEEN

1. Granger Westberg, *Good Grief*, p. 30.

2. Robert Davis, *My Journey into Alzheimer's Disease: A Story of Hope* (Wheaton: Tyndale House, 1989), p. 114.

3. Elisabeth Elliot, *Loneliness* (Nashville: Oliver Nelson, 1988).

CHAPTER FIFTEEN

1. Nancy L. Mace and Peter V. Rabins, *The 36-Hour Day* (New York: Johns Hopkins University Press, Warner Books Edition, 1992), p. 326.

2. For more information about both publications see the Counsel and Care website: www.counselandcare.org.uk

3. See Veterans UK website: http://www.veterans-uk.info/faqs/welfare.html

APPENDIX B

1. Fact sheets on Alzheimer's, various types of chronic dementias and other conditions that can cause dementia can be found on a number of websites; for example, the Alzheimer's Society UK websites and websites of Alzheimer's societies or associations in other countries in the UK and the US. Various associations such as the Parkinson's Disease Society UK, the Huntington's Disease Association UK and the Multiple Sclerosis Society UK also have updated information for carers related to these conditions and dementia.

Index